Grove Health Science Series: Book IV (4)

I0485052

Grove Health Science Series:Book 4
by Joseph & Sari Grove
series edited by Justin Wood

Table of Contents...

If you know the element a flower contains, then you can plant according to your biochemical needs...   **164**

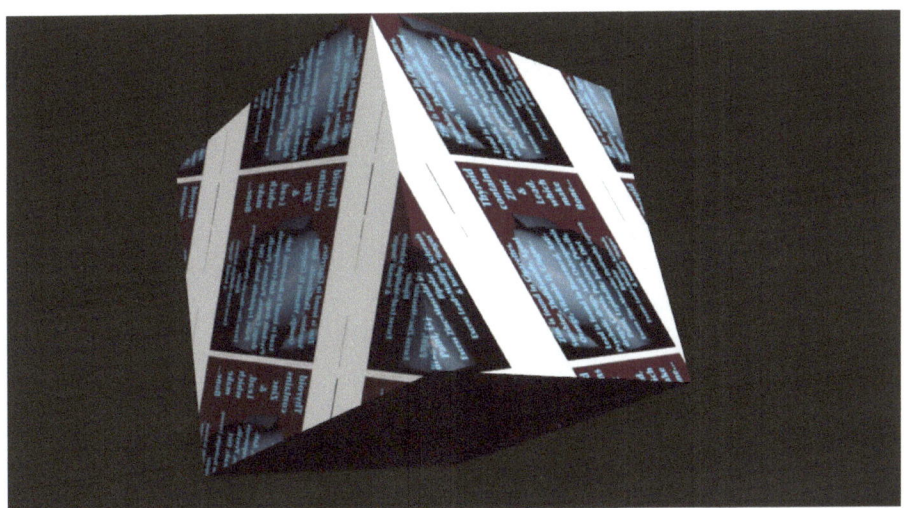

Beforewords...

In Book 3 of this Grove Health Science Series, I embarked on figuring out a nonsurgical answer to getting rid of a breast cancer lump...
I succeeded in figuring out how to turn it from malignant to benign, but needed another book to figure out how to get rid of the lump itself too...
This is pretty hard & complicated work I am doing...
It requires alot of research, alot of thinking, alot of trial & errors...Alot...It is hard...
Figuring out hard things requires much out of the box type thinking...Creative...
The type of thinking an artist does...Which I am, so that is good...
But there is an element of the abstract that occurs when I am solving for something...
Randomness...Crazyness...Yes, I do feel you have to be willing to be crazy in order to come up with the hard answers...
So, like all my books, there are elements of randomness...Things that aren't logical...
I struggle with that...Do I remove the weird stuff from my books?
I cannot...
You won't believe that I came up with the answer if I take away all the evidence...
If it is too perfect it won't be authentic...
Plus, how will you see how I got to something?
As it is it is usually obscure, even to myself...
Anyways...The books are not perfect...I cannot edit the weird out...

I mean, I have been trying to figure out a way for women to get rid of a breast cancer lump...Without going to a doctor...
I think that is a pretty big thing to try to do...
(By the way, I did succeed, but it took me up till Book 6 to nail down a full protocol...Book 6 is short & just gives that protocol...I call it RepoWoman...)
Anyways...
I flit back & forth from the medicine stuff to art then to just other ideas...This helps my brain to relax...
I do eventually get there...Bear with me...
I'm guessing as I get older, my ideas will be more formulated, more perfect sounding, more sure of themselves...
But I will need these early books as witness to how I all got there...
It's important...

Hugs, Sari Grove

Construction worker health problems...

Mastic Glue, Drywall, Wet cement(Sat. July 12, 2014):

As I walked home from Longo's with a giant bag of groceries, I took the library side street, because I was hoping the sad shirtless man with white powder on his face & chest, who was sitting as still as a sculpture, brown-skinned & greying nibs of hair, sitting in front of the Metro Toronto Library as 24 maybe pigeons ate happily in that sunshine, & he with harlequin expression seemed to need me to bring to him one of my newly bought green Granny Smith apples which who possibly could refuse the gift?

But a soccer ball escaped somehow into the street & I saw quickly a boy who might give chase...Knowing that had dangerous consequences, I stuck my arm out to block any particular car who might come by, & dashed & caught the ball with a leg, & deftly kicked it lightly to return it to its young owner, who apparently was most grateful for the interception of events...

As I walked by the carwash where the boy's father owned & worked, another 2 men glared at me with thanks...One said in a thick accent:"The score is 2 nothing"...Then:"Netherlands Brazil"...I had no idea what he was talking about, but apparently I was getting the scores on something as a thank you..."What?" I said..."What are you talking about?"...
"In the soccer...Fifa...In the soccer match"...
Oh, I laughed loud..."I'M A GIRL!!!"...
I explained that I was happily grocery shopping, though my husband was glued to some flatscreen tv set in a bar with a bunch of losers & winners who were all also nursing mediocre draft beer & rather good chicken wings while seemingly all pretending to care deeply about the soccer...

My husband confessed to me this afternoon he still ponders why he watched the World Cup Soccer year after year, though he has yet to understand how it can touch others & him mostly bored but trying to feel the touch...(I said:"why don't you stop? Like when I finally stopped trying to enjoy pot-smoking in university despite everyone's suggestion that it was such a good time...It just made my lips dry & then I was unable to have the meaningful kind of conversations I enjoyed having in university settings...)

But back to my newfound friends at the Carwash...In the course of light banter between people who are trying to say thank you & me who just generally loves meeting new & unique humans & animals & plants & such, I usually early on give someone one of my neat business cards, with my Grove Body Part Chart on the back, & a website address to read my books for free on their home computer...

GROVE BODY PART CHART

Read our book

Grove Body Part Chart:A Medical Arts Innovation

online as a free pdf embed on our website...

www.grovecanada.ca

by Joseph & Sari Grove
grove@sent.com

Each Organ has 2 opposing elements, that live in balance...

Organ	Minus Element	Plus Element
Thyroid	Zinc	Lead
Thymus	Manganese	Iron
Lungs & Lymph Nodes	Titanium	Aluminum
Heart	Potassium	Aurum
Kidneys	Carbon	Nitrogen
Pancreas	Selenium	Sulphur
Liver	Oxygen	Hydrogen
Adrenal Gland	Iodine	Calcium
Spleen	Copper	Phosphorus
Gallbladder	Magnesium	Mercury
Colon	Fluorine	Bismuth

Grove Body Part Chart

Here are the 2 sides to one of our early business cards, the one for the first book about our chart idea, called "Grove Body Part Chart:A Medical Arts Innovation"...

People always read the front of the card first, so I tend to lean forward & turn it over to show them the chart, so I can explain how it works on the spot..."See, there are 11 organs, & in each organ there are 2 elements that live together as opposites"...

Then I usually get a question about something that is usually tricky..."What about blood circulation" one man said..."Well, blood is made in the Thymus gland, which is made of Iron & Manganese..."
"Magnesium?" the man said..."No Manganese...Magnesium is in the gallbladder..."
"You find Manganese in nuts, all nuts...Nuts lower iron..."

Satisfied with my answer, the man asks:"What about bone marrow?"...But then, he decides that he knows the answer & starts talking about his life & his story...
As I type this out this evening, it occurs to me that the white stuff in bone marrow would be Phosphorus, & the red stuff blood...But the white, well more a little yellow stuff would be Phosphorus, & that is made by the Spleen & its opposite is Copper...But I digress...

The man tells me that in 1992 he had a pain in his right ankle...Wouldn't go away...Went to doctors & specialists, then more doctors & more specialists, & nobody could tell him why he had pain in his right ankle...

Then he said one night he woke up & it seemed like the skin had peeled off from his toes on the right foot...Scared, no terrified, he went back to all the doctors & specialists...One suggested he get an angiogram...A heart circulation blood circulation type test...Ah...This was why he was interested in blood...

The specialist, probably a cardiologist (though he didn't say his English was a bit raw, he was Turkish I think...) The specialist said the man had diabetes, high blood sugar, in the P-A-N-C-R-E-A-S...

The man was not happy with this diagnosis...The toes episode was gangrene...Gangrene is a worst case scenario with untreated diabetes...He was given drugs & such...The man then went to the States where a I think maybe a Naturopath type doctor gave the man a bevy of vitamins to take...The man was not really impressed with that so much either...

So the man somehow found this Muslim Turkish man, who had studied in Turkey, a technique called blood cupping...For $50.00 every 2 months, from 2009 to 2013, the man went to this person for a blood cupping session...

The first session, the blood that came out was like jelly...Jelly-like...

Apparently the blood cupping was done ALL OVER this man's body at different times...His head...His back...His legs...All over...

The second or third session, the blood came out in places black...I told him this was the gangrenous blood coming out...Gangrene...yes he said he knew...

Then finally after he said maybe 36 cups over time had been taken from him, the blood finally came out a normal true red colour & normal runny consistency...

It was alot of blood & I cautioned him to be careful if he felt cured not to continue with this treatment in fear that he might overdo the process...

But he said he felt fine, not lacking in energy, in fact he had more energy, & that he alot of goat & some other animal I couldn't hear the word properly, but that he was eating very well on purpose, I heard liver as well, to boost his system...

He told me in one of the blood cupping sessions, the practitioner(for want of a better word here?) had done work on the man's right calf at the back...

Blood Cupping

The blood cupping he explained was like this: The man would put a suction cup on the area until it maybe even turned a little purple, then the man would scratch the surface of the area very very lightly with a needle or even a razor, then put the suction cup back on to suck out the blood there...

In one critical session, the back of his calf session-the practitioner had found & removed a sugar cube sized thing from the back of the man's calf...This had been stuck there & was what was causing the pain for so many years...

I asked:"Why was your body so full of sugar???" "I mean, what caused this sugar excess problem?"...(Note:Sugar is a Sulphur excess in the pancreas which can be antidoted by adding Seleniums to the diet like raw garlic or spicy hot habenero peppers or garlic pills...Medically Seleniums are in insulin & antibiotics...Quinine is a selenium you can get in Tonic water..."

The man said...I am an immigrant, so I worked in construction...We were exposed to mastic glue in the wet cement, to drywall, all sorts of toxic chemicals...

Yes I thought to myself, glues & turpentines can mimic Hydrogens & Sulphurs, which can muck up your Liver & your Pancreas especially...I myself take garlic if I have a paint headache, & Goji berries(high in Oxygen content) help me when I have a glue headache...(I was making homemade marble which required alot of glue as a binder for the marble powder)...

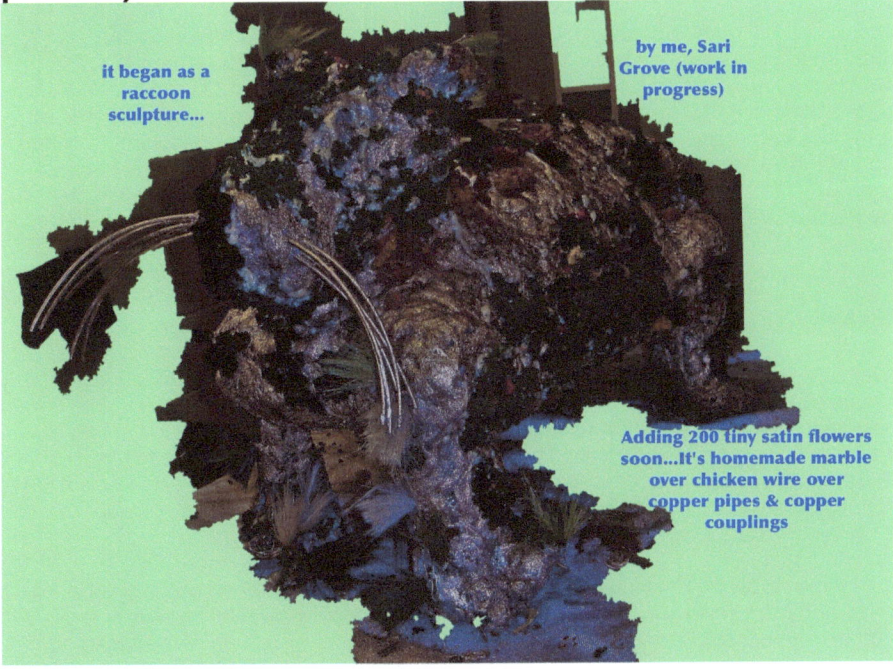

it began as a raccoon sculpture...

by me, Sari Grove (work in progress)

Adding 200 tiny satin flowers soon...It's homemade marble over chicken wire over copper pipes & copper couplings

the picture shows the in progress work on the raccoon sculpture in marble...You can see my finished works & recipes for marble & concrete & no-weld armature designs on our website at
http://www.grovecanada.ca

(yes it looks more like a dog...Unfortunately the raccoon had been hit by a car & I was unable to reconstruct his jaw in my mind or in reality because it had been so damaged by the car...

So the sculpture morphed a bit as my Mother's Portuguese Water Dog became a substitute model...I am an abstract artist at heart, which means I am comfortable with things not looking like reality, plus I don't work from photographs which means I do the best I can from looking at something or from memory, but if that fails me I really try hard to NOT use photos as reference...I feel the so-called flaw in the sculpture causes the story to be told...

Had I "fixed" the sculpture by using photos of raccoons to reconstruct the jaw, there would be no question as to why it was referred to as a raccoon sculpture though it looked like a dog...I like the flaws...I learned this as a child when my mother explained to me that carpet maker artists put flaws in their carpets on purpose so as not to offend God with their feelings that their work was so perfect...Animals are made not to be exactly the same on each side of a carpet...Like that...It is a form of humility I respect & have grown up to try to emulate a bit...Realism in art tends to upset me slightly for that reason...

The man at the Carwash wanted to continue his story, but I felt it was time to give my green freshly bought Granny Smith apple to the man at the Library who had looked so sad & I said as much & left with a "Bye" & a smile to the boy & his soccer ball...

It is 10:16 pm tonight, a Saturday night in July, & my husband is out at the bar again, & though my heart aches a tiny little bit with loneliness at his being not here with me, it does help me to work...When he is away I get my work done...When he is home, I sit near him & do not as much of anything, just whatever it takes to be close to him...My husband comes from the "hard-to-get" school of husbands & apparently that type does not quit once the marriage vows get said...He is still hard to get, so I still pursue, though it may seem like idiocy as we are nearing our 18th year of marriage...

But I think I have begun this 4th book well...The man at the carwash had a good story one worthy to be told in a book, of a problem that may be sadly more common to people who work in construction than we know...This blood cupping technique is interesting medically & the man said he would give the healer who did this for him a million dollars if he could for saving his life...I am glad this man is well...It makes me happy when I have no advice to give...

Truth is one of my goals in writing my books was to help people to heal so nobody I knew would be sick anymore so we could all just be happy & go out & play...yes, I am a child...I just want to play...I get so bored of people being too sick to play with me...If every could just get well soon, we could all get back to the real work of play!!!

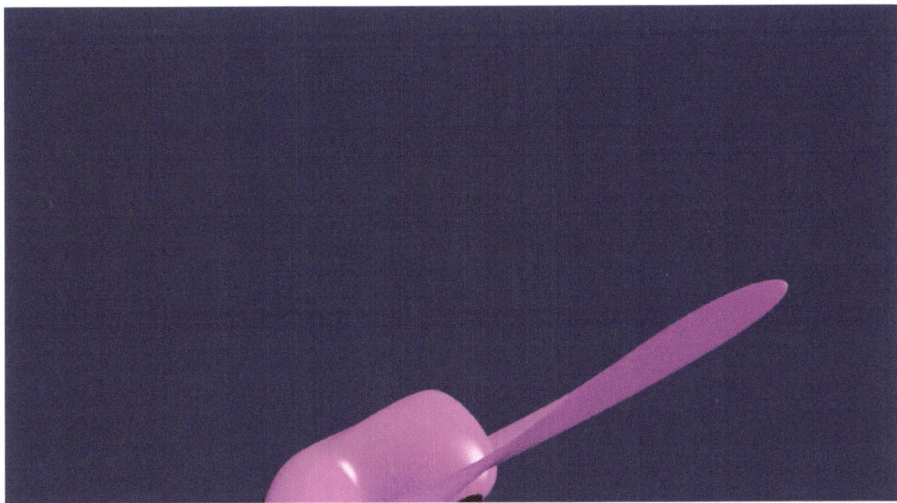

http://www.fightthenewdrug.org/ I was reading an article in the Huffington Post about a 59 year old woman with a great body whose new boyfriend wouldn't sleep with her because she was too wrinkly...Commenters mentioned that older men today have such access to porn that it creates unrealistic perceptions that a 22 year old porn star is actually a feasible mate...That the older female is no longer attractive enough...Though I am perhaps not militant about porn, I think this is an interesting idea to ponder...This organization seems to be working on this idea & has some interesting statistics...Personally I think free porn accessibility, from an artist's perspective, means that the "artists" so to speak are not getting paid...I have a problem with artists not getting paid...On the other hand, when things are not lucrative people tend to find other jobs, so maybe that is a good thing? Don't know, still on the fence about all of this...I do know that it is all fine if I do it, but if my husband does it it is a heinous crime...But that's how I see everything! LOL!

http://yourbrainonporn.com/ Your brain on porn has more information about addiction & this phenomenon today...

http://pornharms.com/ Porn harms is another such site along the same lines as the first 2...

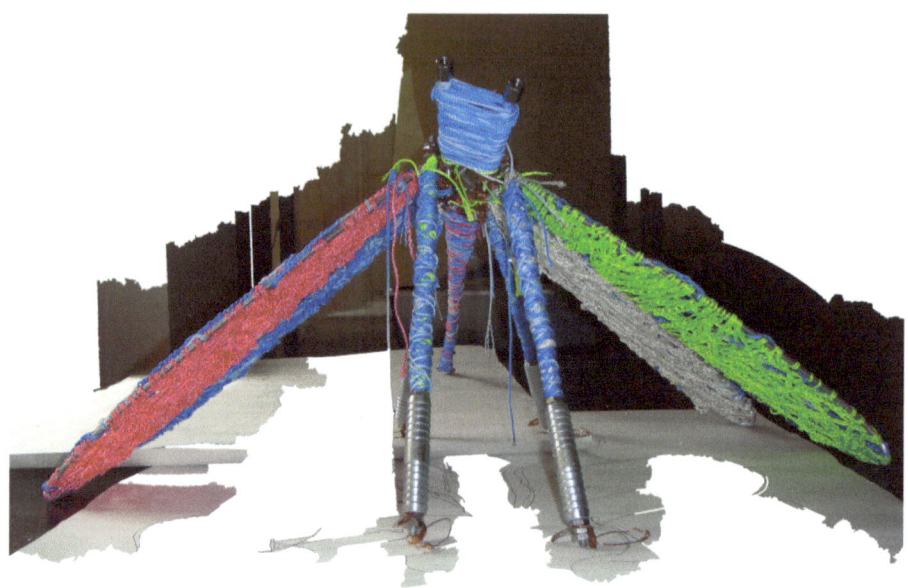

Dragonfly is made of an original no-weld armature design by Sari Grove that uses plumber's copper strapping, bolts & threaded steel rods, with hand knotted Mason's brick line nylon cord for the wings...All the parts are moveable...Dragonfly was featured in a beautiful art show at the restored PaperMill(yes it was an old Paper Mill & they made it so nice! & added a theatre too!) Gallery in Toronto, Ontario, Canada...The show was called "Childsight" & it was about how children perceive things...To me, bugs have always been giants...My Essence of Bee sculpture was also huge...

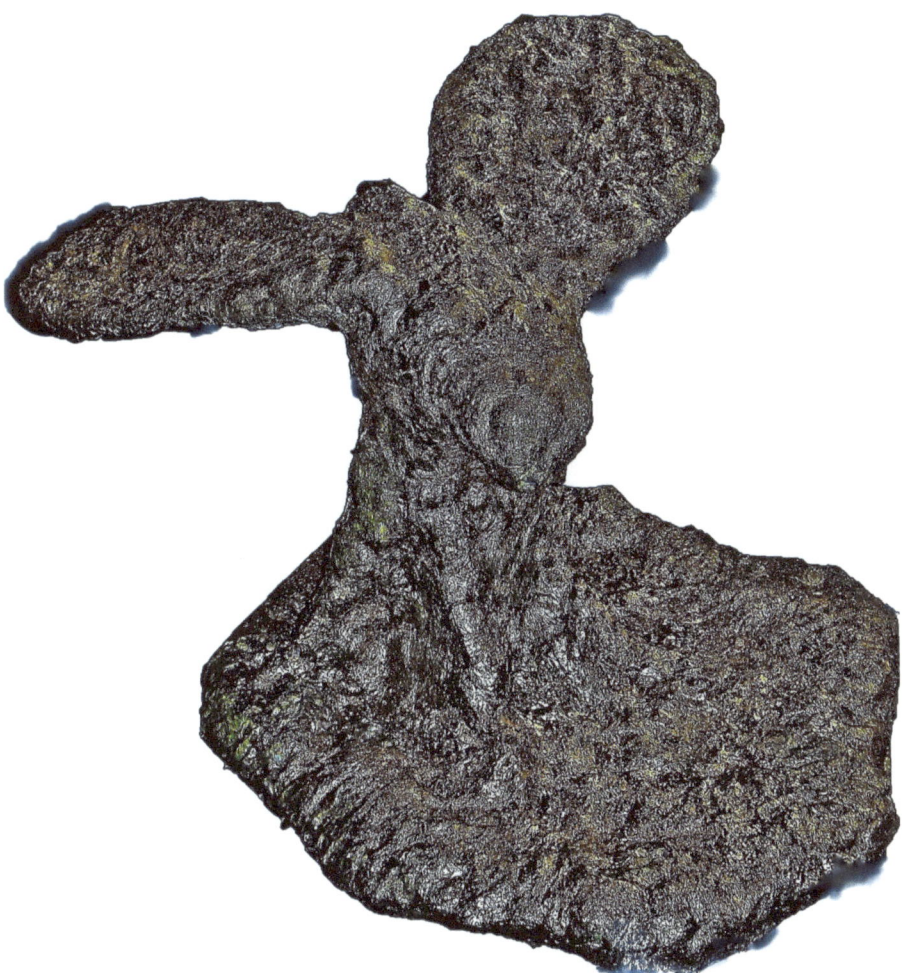

Essence of Bee by Sari Grove is about 2 feet by 3 feet by 2 feet, think of a breadbox maybe or bigger, made of Sari's Concrete recipe but modified to add way more Aragonite sand which is actually a marble sand...The extra marble sand makes it far softer & more pliable...While the marble concrete was still wet, Sari brushed in real gold powder mixed with a natural Dammar varnish to give it the gold sheen...Essence of bee lives happily in a garden outside in the Forest Hill area of Toronto...Inside is the no-weld armature design Sari invented to hold steel rods together without having to undergo the burn dangers of welding...

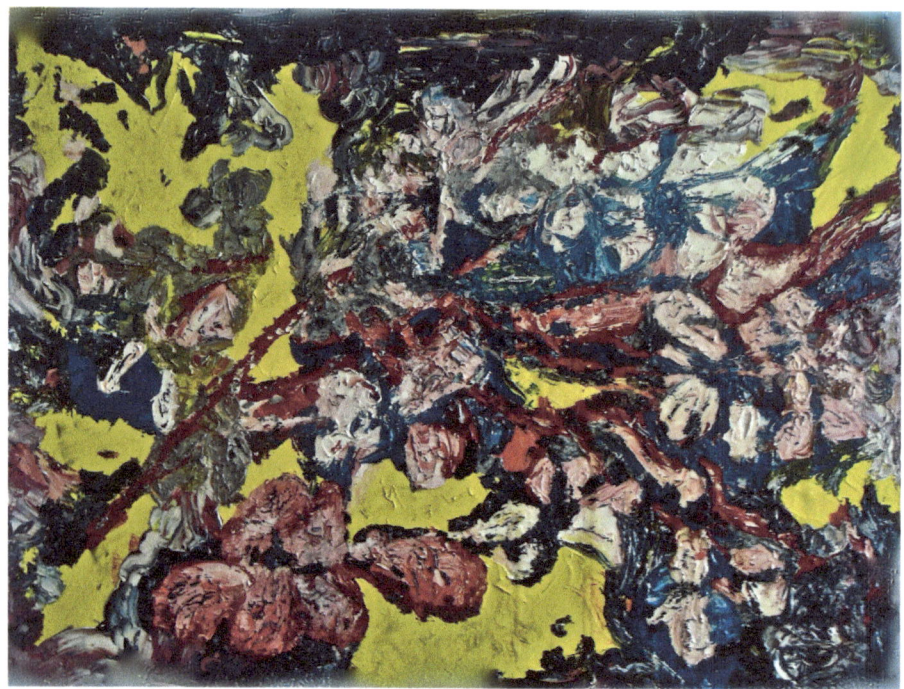

Magnolia is a 3 foot by 4 foot walnut oil painting by Sari Grove circa 2011-about 6 months of work...It was painted with a knife using both the left & right hand...It sits on a belgian linen cloth at 10 weight...Coated with natural Dammar varnish that uses no turpentines, but instead a citrus solvent based on orange juice...Stretcher bars are made of basswood which is sustainable & grows quickly...Jimmy Carter used to grow Paulownia trees which are similar to basswood in sustainability, & grow quickly...

About how this book is going to go...

In my last year at McGill University I had to fill in some course requirements...I think I was short in the Literature department...The only course I could find that could fit into my schedule, which included not taking courses that were too early in the morning because in Montreal some mornings the snow was 4 feet deep & even though I lived close to McGill it could still take me half an hour to walk to class through the snowdrifts & I would inevitable be late...By my last year of school I had learned this the hard way, so by then I was only choosing classes that began after 10:30 am in the morning...I still was often late & grew to understand that lateness was just part of my character...Though the few times in my life that I had been the early bird I did get the worm so to speak...Must remember that lesson & apply that more often...Perhaps this old dog can learn a new trick???

Anyways, sigh...I took a course in Faulkner...William Faulkner...We were studying the Sound & the Fury first...I was excited...This was going to be revelatory...Then I read the Sound & the Fury...I was bored...I didn't get it...I re-read it...Nothing nada nothing...Didn't get the greatness of it...Was I an idiot?

I went home for Christmas was it? Asked my Dad...Dad, why is the Sound & the Fury such a great book? I don't get it...Why?

My Dad answered...:" because he was the first person to record, write down, what the people in the South were saying...Their speech...The content...He wrote it down...prior to then, everybody thought the people were just speaking gibberish...

That they were stupid...After Faulkner's book people realized that the folk were actually speaking English, just a pidgeon English with variations, a dialect of sorts, but that those "folk" so to speak were definitely not stupid, in fact to the contrary, highly intelligent...This moved those "folk" forward indescribably in time...(We are referring to African Americans here-but my Dad didn't label things much, he knew I knew what he was talking about...My Dad was very polite that way...Canadians tend to be polite about things-you probably know that already...)

So...Anyways...Long story short, Faulkner was great because he listened to people & then wrote down what they said...He listened to people who hadn't been listened to before...& wrote it down...Sort of translated their speech...

I was thinking for this 4th book in our series-Grove Health Science Series:Book 4, that maybe I would listen to people who hadn't been listened to before...& write it down...Sort of translate a bit...So maybe this book will incorporate interview stories with real people who I will meet in my daily walks...I've been walking about 10 kilometres here or there as often as I can...In my third book Algae+Rhythm, Algae-Rhyme:Apt surgical rotation app I talk about my efforts to get rid of a breast lump...This is when I started walking far in a more serious & regular way...I always have walked, & talked to people as I walked, but it is more part of my life now...So why not use these conversations as fodder for this book? I am not Faulkner, but why not try that idea? It is maybe not original anymore, but I think the concept still has legs...Besides, Canadians are still mostly an unexamined sort-this might be useful...

I bet my newfound & quickly lost(we live in different sectors of the city & I am not good with date commitments) ephemeral friend the radical anthropologist might be interested...

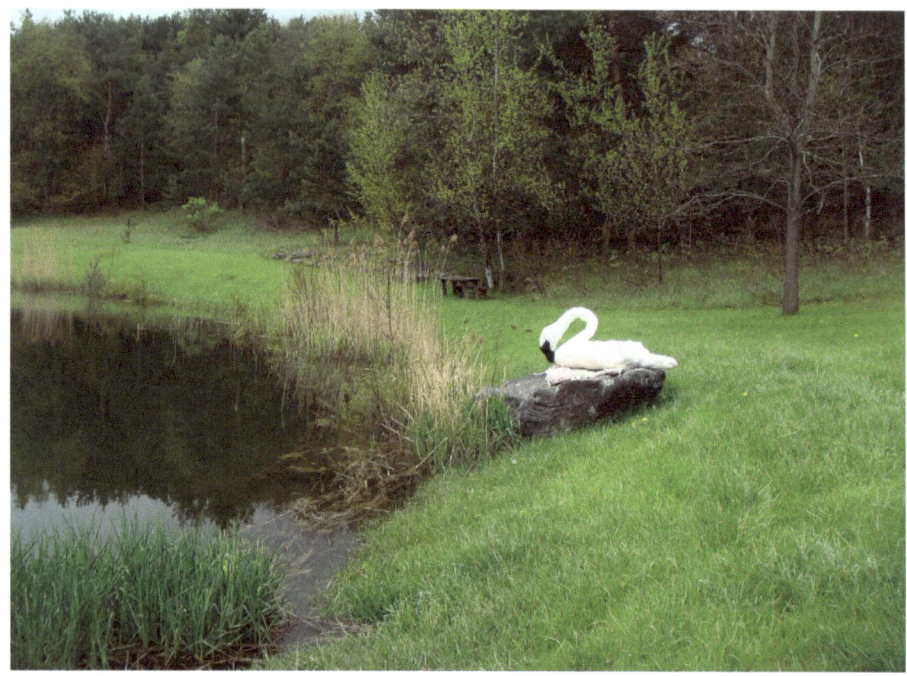

Swanee is over a year's worth of effort learning concrete & armatures & it is maybe 5 feet long & weights over 100 lbs & it is of a Trumpeter swan & sits North & West of Toronto, about 45 minutes driving time, near a pond, on a private farm, on a Trumpeter swan flight path...The concrete recipe sari invented for this work was designed especially to withstand very harsh climactic conditions...The recipe is on her website for those working in cold harsh conditions...

After 3 years, the sculpture is holding up well...It is also attracting all sorts of waterbirds & earth birds as well as humans & dogs & deer & the horses like it too as well as the trees...The hand knotted nest underneath has faded to a muslin colour but that actually looks better than the original reds greens & yellows turns out...The artificial nest for a swan design instructions are on Instructables as well as on Sari's website...(again at http://www.grovecanada.ca)

Epilepsy:

On one of my 10 km walks, right at the end, as I made my way up the very steep hill, & a bicyclist struggled with me, almost at the same pace it was so steep...

We made it to the top & both exclaimed with some sort of a grunt or sigh of relief...

We walked together for a while as we cooled down from our respective workouts...

As we chatted, the subject of medicine came up, of course...

The man, a father, told me of his son, who at age 6 started having seizures...
The father took him to a specialist who recommended heavy anti-epileptic medication...
The father then went to a Chinese doctor who interestingly advised the father to massage his son's feet at night & watch & wait & see...
The boy who is now in his 20s, & has completed university, is fine & has been seizure free for 14 years...
The father had faithfully done the nightly foot massage on his son's feet...
The seizures never came back touch wood...
It was a good story...

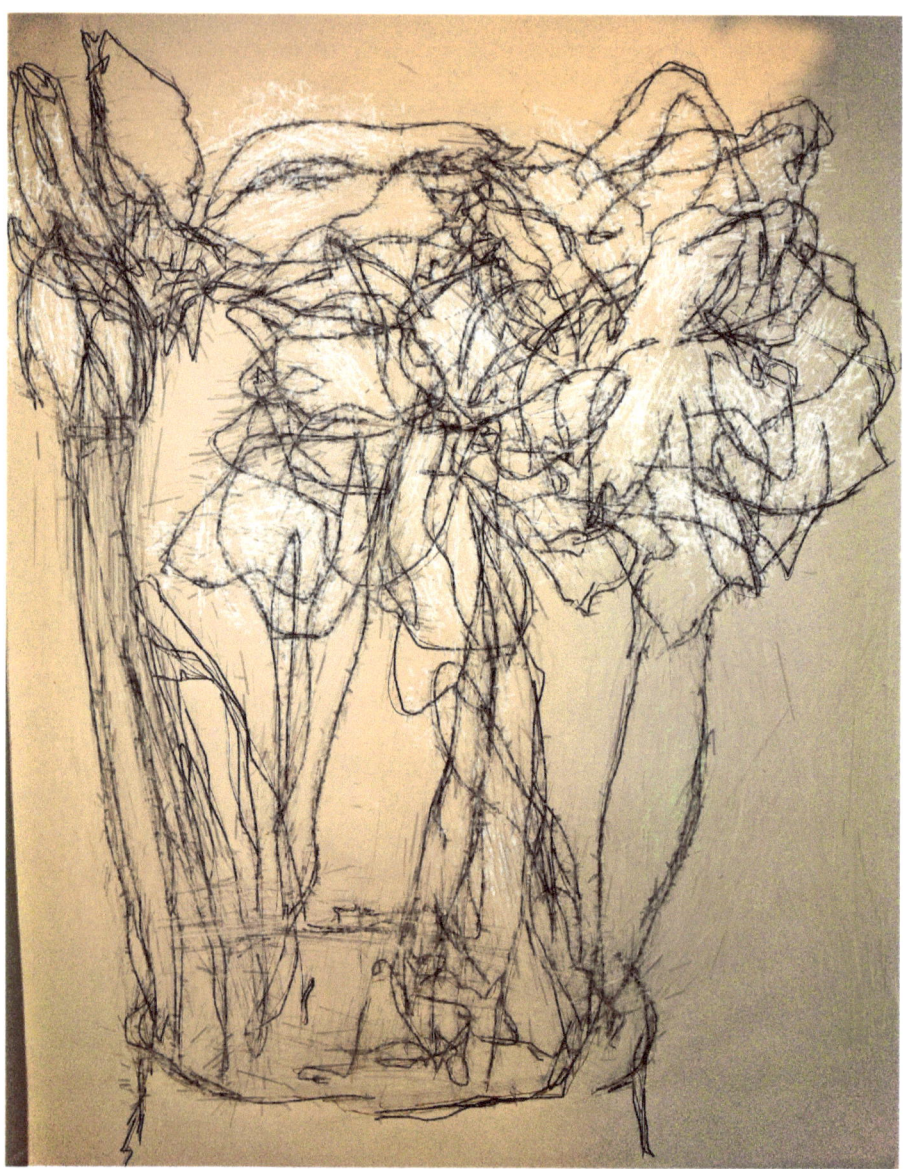

Amaryllis is a from life drawing of real blooming Amaryllis bulbs, by Sari Grove about 30 inches wide by 40 inches tall, on paper, drawn in black pen...It was later photographed

& uploaded to a computer, then the black lines were drawn over with computer pen to make them appear darker...Then some white lines were scumbled(sort of scratched in) also using the computer pen program, to show the flowers were white...This was made into a poster & printed out...

Degenerating Spinal Discs:

A woman was told that her spinal discs were degenerating & if she did not have surgery she would in the future be crippled...

The woman, at the age of maybe 37 & a half, weighed a mere 123 lbs. at 5' 6" or maybe 5' 7" I am guessing here...(though the weight is accurate)...

The woman who had once been a dancer, was also a vegetarian coming into 30 years as such...

Two other habits were pertinent...1)Mode of transportation was a self-built bicycle which was used continuously including for social events & career appointments, no matter if the event was one hour away & up hills the whole entire way...

2) Favorite hangout was a biker coffee bar where the coffee was about as strong as you could get-meaning it makes Starbucks look like dishwater strong...

Comment:Discs in the spine are bendy & move & are connected by cartilage...One of the fastest ways to boost cartilage is by upping your Bilirubin levels...This is in the gallbladder...Since a vegetarian won't eat pork for the added mercury benefit(pork raises bilirubin quickly helping to rebuild cartilage & tendons), the cheap solution is to add SALT to the diet...Alot of salt...This will make a skinny over-exercising person retain water...The water-retention actually helps to serve as a nutrient in the body, feeding the starving parts...

Over-exercising is a sure way to degenerate discs, & all cartilage in general...Cut that out!

Coffee is often full of magnesium which lowers bilirubin sometimes dangerously...The magnesium in coffee can cause over-poohing, then hemorrhoids, then severe back pain & things people may call Sciatica...It is actually the sciatic nerve that gets stripped when you pooh too much from getting too much magnesium in your diet or exercising too much...Coffee's primary ingredient is copper but watch out-magnesium sneaks in sometimes in cheaper brands...The coffee will taste good but will have too much of a laxative effect...If you get a sore neck after drinking coffee that is magnesium...Sometimes more expensive coffees are mostly copper & less magnesium...Cheaper coffee brands like the Tim Horton's brand, tastes good, is cheap, but is way more magnesium & way less copper...

Last bit: Generally speaking in the case of too skinny, exercises too much, strict restrictive diet & very low body weight, the most general thing you can say is to gain some weight like at least 10 pounds, plus start expanding your vegetarian diet with maybe some supplements or a strong multivitamin...Theoretically you can avoid spinal surgery but you really have to want to gain some weight...You can't stay dancer skinny & expect your body to repair damage...

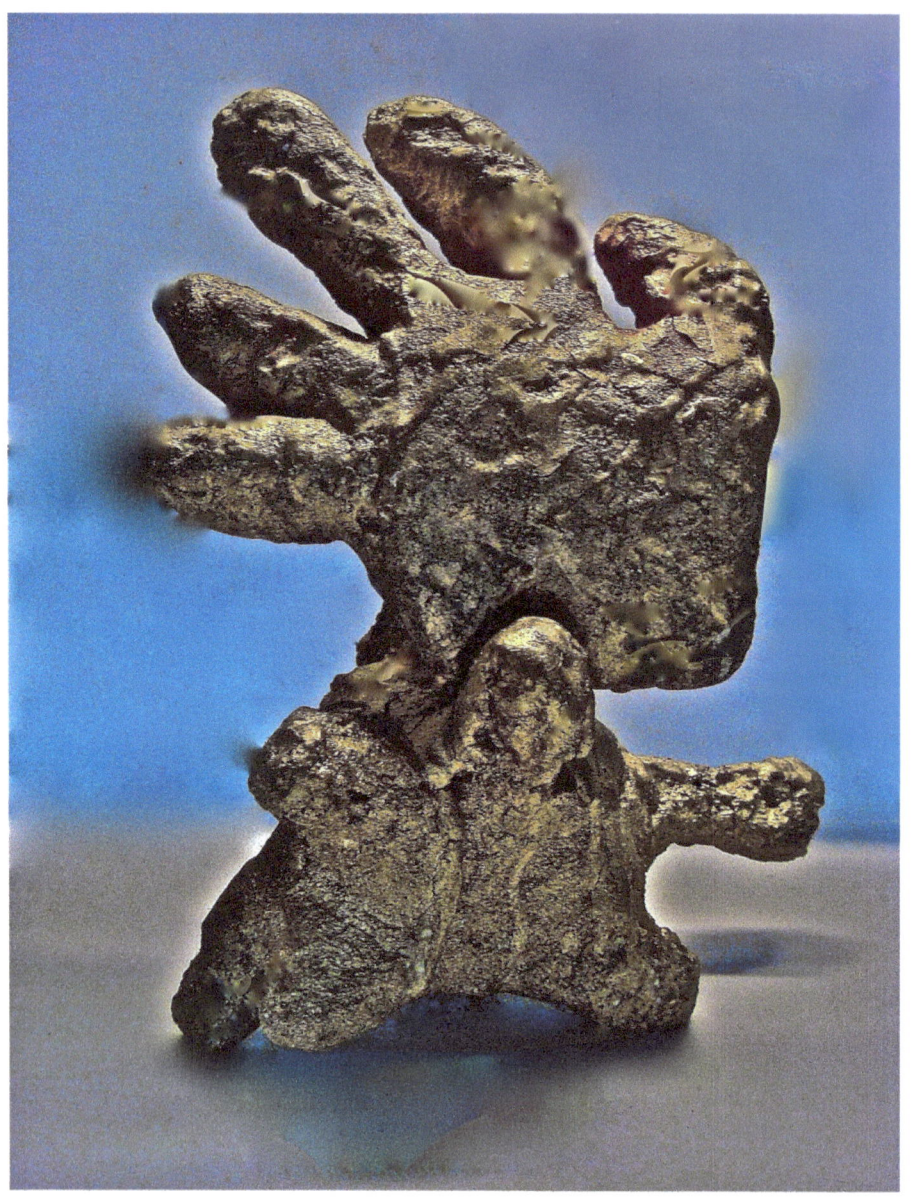

The picture above shows a figure carrying another figure on its back...These are 2 separate sculptures made of steel rods armatures, held with bolts & screws & copper strapping, covered in aluminum screening, tied on with copper wire, then covered with my own homemade marble mixture which includes Aragonite sand, glues, 3/4" alkaline resistant glass fibres, real gold powder, dammar varnish, & silicon sand-oh & water...

This was actually an early prototype for a prosthetic left hand, which, when the metal parts became too heavy, got covered in the marble & turned into a sculpture instead...A later prototype was much lighter & less hand-like in appearance...The base was actually a piece I called War Toy which looked like an earlier bronze piece I had made that was based on an abstract blowfish...When it got covered also in marble it became blobbier & took on character...

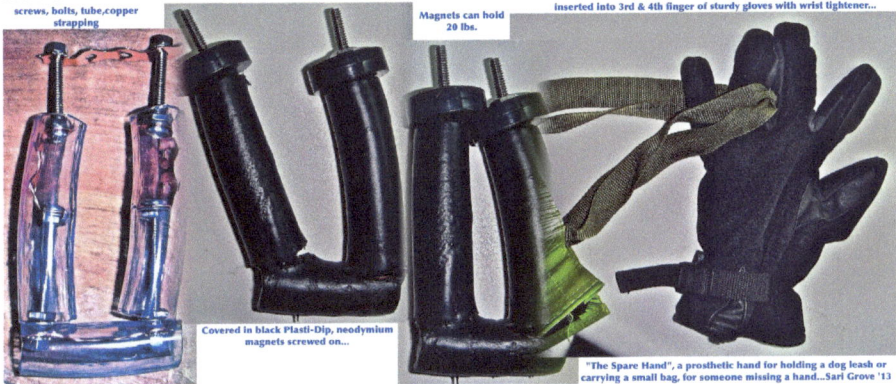

The "finished" prosthetic became more of a clutch piece based on magnets...When you put the clutch into a glove it becomes handlike in appearance & can be used for casual outings quickly, like walking the dog to hold the leash, or carrying a grocery bag...For times when a heavier regular prosthetic is too much...A strong wrist strap on a glove would be helpful, to hold the glove to the end of the arm...This is a far as I could go on this concept, & I am sure the next artist or designer could use it & take it further...I put the project aside, since my brain was tired for just getting to there...I may pick up the project again if I get any newer ideas coming my way in that direction...

http://didhemaketheputt.com Did he make the putt, is a website that follows after the film called Utopia, which is about improving your golf game & then improving your life...It is buried in a sports psychology movie but springs forth with God's own truths...No way else to say it...It is powerful as most Robert Duvall films are...

Recipe:

When I finally broke through with my discovery about breast cancer's nature & then subsequently was able to stop it in its tracks(read Book 3 of this series to see how that all happened-the book is called Algae+Rhythm, Algae-Rhyme:Apt Surgical Rotation App), I was also helped by changing my diet drastically that particular week in time...I switched to a mostly all raw vegetable diet, though I did "cheat" a bit with fish since I am usually a dizzy if I only eat vegetables...

Here is the salad that served as the backdrop to my using licorice(powder, capsules, tea, tincture-they are all pretty good in different ways though really watch the alcohol with the tincture-sometimes the tinctures arrive all alcohol & not much licorice for some reason)...

Sari's salad:Let's be honest, the ingredients are all up in the air, just mess around with them & improvise & add more of what you like & skip what you don't like...

Green Apples big pieces
Walnuts
Sunflower seeds
Some sort of salad green like baby spinach
Maybe some cabbage
Maybe some kale
Maybe some shredded brussel sprouts
Shredded almonds
Dried cranberries
Pumpkin seeds
Poppy seeds
An avocado in pieces
Maybe an organic carrot in large pieces or even shredded
Ok I cheat & add either a water packed high quality dolphin free can of tuna, or
My other cheat is a tin of smoked mussels with or without the oily liquid

Now the salad dressing is key:

Apple Cider Vinegar (I actually use a clearer one than Bragg's though most people swear by Bragg's)
Really high quality Olive Oil (the one I use has that skinny pour spout attached to the top so you can drizzle if you want)
Squeeze a whole lemon with your hands(if you squeeze the lemon over the other hand you can catch the seeds before it goes into whatever you are putting the lemon juice into)
Dijon Horseradish Mustard (a really generous glob or two)

Honestly I began by putting all the ingredients for the dressing into a shakey bottle with a lid & shaking, but recently found it was just fine to dump each ingredient one at a time into the salad & just stir the whole thing well after...

Let the salad rest in the fridge or wherever for a while for the flavours to set in better...

Ok that's it! That's the salad that gave me tons of energy while cleansing out my system, while I was taking licorice root in various forms to turn my breast lump from malignant to benign...

To be honest, it was CRUCIAL to switch to a raw vegetable diet while fixing this breast lump to be benign...

With the almost daily 10 kilometer walks in the sun on a dirt trail...(Teva Hurricane hiking sandals are awesome, have good treads for arch support, & you can rinse them daily with water to get the dirt out-$35 on sale on Amazon one fine day...)

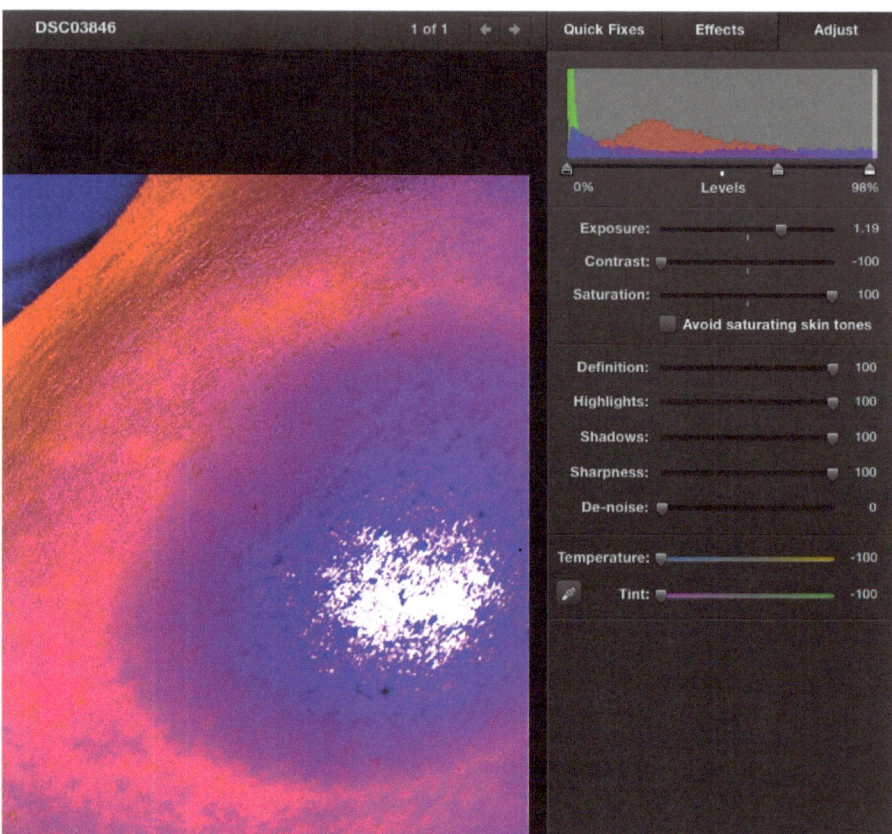

(Morning of July 14, 2014-after I made the mistake of using a Poppyseed pre-fab salad dressing the night before which had sugar in it...)The picture above shows my left mammary gland(breast), cropped for modesty...The shiny white reflective thing is calcium oxalate...A calcium Oxalate lump is a benign lump made of calcium & iron (oxalate)...The tiny purple/navy specks are Phosphorus...A calcium Phosphate (Phosphorus) lump is malignant...breast cancer, DCIS(ductal cancer in situ) whatever you want to call it...Dangerous possibly...Phosphorus in excess is the same thing that you get when you get Salmonella poisoning...It is a creeping mold type thing...In fact if you look at a Salmonella bacterium & a calcium Phosphate lump up close, they look alike...Sort of like purple ants...

Notice in the (the lump pic.)picture:The photo was taken with a Sony DSC-T100 point & shoot no external lens 8 megapixel digital camera, on Macro, with Flash on, held close to my left breast, from the side, where the lump is...Uploaded to a mac Snow leopard computer desktop, into iPhoto, in the Edit mode, Boosted 9 times(all the way) in Effects, then in the Adjust section just see the settings where they are in the Photo...(I used the Grab program to capture my computer screen so you could see the Adjust settings, so you could try doing a Mammogram or other Digital-Gram at home yourself with your own camera...)

below handpainted by Sari pic shows Salmonella (my image was inspired by this scanning electron micrograph from Auburn University Veterinary medicine school http://www.vetmed.auburn.edu/salmonella#.U8PO828e1bw)

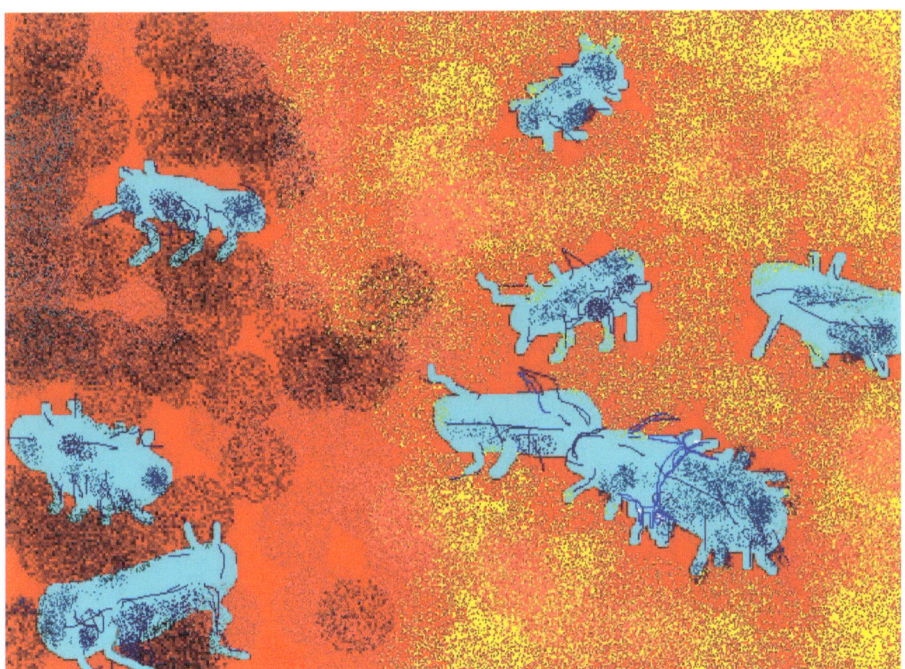

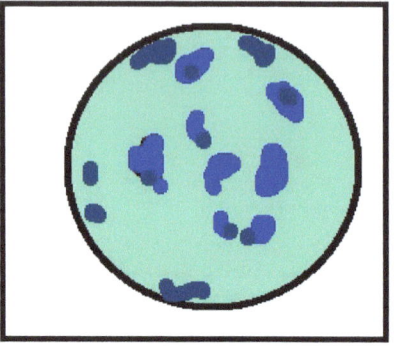

Calcium Phosphate(Malignant

Phosphorus is what makes a lump

cancer...

Licorice(a Copper) lowers

Phosphorus...

　*spatial light interference microscopy (SLIM)

　**Tissue refractive index as marker of disease

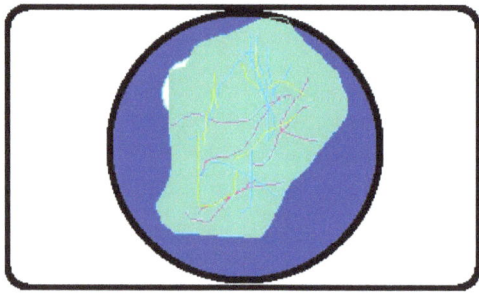

Calcium Oxalate(benign)

In Spectral Light Interference Microscopy(SLIM),

a malignant lump(Calcium Phosphorus) looks like the same Salmonella creatures

in the previous picture
(like purple ants
-though in the electron scan micrograph the
 purple ants come out like turquoise ants
-ironically,
 or coincidentally, or, really,
 turquoise, the stone from Arizona,
 is a Phosphorus stone-
so the electron scan micrograph colour
 is probably truer in colour nature to real)...
Which stands to reason, because Both Salmonella bacteria & Calcium Phosphate
malignant breast cancer lumps contain PHOSPHORUS...(which spreads like mold
which is how cancer gets called INVASIVE, like mold...)

If breast cancer(Calcium Phosphate lump) is in fact a salmonella bacterium spreading(a Phosphorus creature), then of course, ingesting say Licorice powder in your tea or coffee would be a nice absorbable strong Copper item that should kill or dissolve those Phosphorus loving creatures...Copper will starve them out...

I write Licorice Powder because it absorbs fast, is a great strong Copper, is relatively cheap & easy to buy, it tastes pretty good in coffee or tea, & isn't too weird, & is an accepted medicine in particular to Hungarians where licorice grows well &,
 by the way did you know Deprenyl the anti-Parkinson's drug was invented in Hungary & is based on licorice & did you know Parkinson's disease was excess Phosphorus in the Spleen usually caused by traumatic injury to the Spleen like getting hit by a streetcar when you were 8 years old in Toronto...

Background:A benevolent well-meaning butcher put out a giant trough of leftover raw meat in a public park in Rosedale...The raccoons & the mice feasted...It was a joyous time...But after 13 days in the park, the trough attracted Salmonella bacteria...Some of the raccoons ate the spoiled meat & got Salmonella poisoning...The raccoon family, 3, tried to wash off in the river by the trail of Milkman's Run, which runs behind the big houses & runners know it...But...
Delusional after a few days, the father raccoon got hit by a car one night under the Crescent street bridge over Mount Pleasant road...A few days later the mom raccoon got hit on Rosedale Valley Road going South...The daughter raccoon was struck a week later on Moore Avenue while going east towards Bayview...
I found the father raccoon first & wrapped him in my very very long merino cashmere sweater carefully without touching him directly, & rested him on my bike seat with one hand while rolling the bike to the Veterinary Emergency Clinic on Yonge street...
R.I.P. ...3 days later I got some strange sort of thing which I thought maybe was lice...Later I thought it was raccoon roundworm...Now I know it was related to a Salmonella bacterium, after many months, no years of investigating what happened in my neighbourhood to cause this tragedy...
3 years later I have a mostly calcium oxalate lump in my left breast which just appeared around Easter 2014, but I see there is some Phosphorus in it, which indicates salmonella bacteria...I am taking Licorice(Copper) as the cure & daily photographing the lump to see how the "ants" in the DIY mammogram are disappearing...& they are hurrah!
I am also on a mainly raw vegetable diet & am taking an Anti-parasitic Cleanse kit of capsules which is a 3 part kit made by Knowledge Products (which I bought at Gingko health Supplement store under Holt Renfrew's on Bloor street, for about $75 Canadian currency)...
So breast cancer is really just Salmonella bacteria is my hunch here considering the past 3 ears of fighting a parasite that I know came from spoiled raw meat ingestion...

By the way:"How did I know about the spoiled raw meat in the park?"...I was investigating the neighbourhood where a raccoon family might go...near to the park is a house...I suspected that house owner would know about wildlife in the park...While loitering near the house I smelled the familiar smell of lead/graphite pencil shavings, lots

of them...(I am an artist, plus I have a really good nose for smells)...I loitered some more & sure enough a person appeared, the owner of the house...
I asked him:"Are you some sort of an artist? I smell pencil shavings..."
He laughed:"Yes, I write children's books...In French...I am french..."
We switched to french for a bit then switched back to English...(thank you Toronto French School for my education up to grade 6 in all french for that!)
He said he uses pencil to sketch out his drawings...(I am guessing the shavings go out his back window into his back garden, which is why I was smelling it all airborne...)
He talked about the mice that lived in his back garden with love, so I knew he liked animals & would do them no harm...
I told him a little about the raccoon family & that I was trying to understand how they got hit by cars-seeing as our Toronto born raccoons are pretty smart, & the downtown ones know about cars usually at night & a whole family was alot to be accidental...
I thought maybe the raccoons were suicidal, as many animals become when sick, but I couldn't figure out what could have made them feel sick enough for that...
(I once saw an injured butterfly in Mexico flying on purpose into a chlorinated pool & decided that even butterflies commit suicide rather than live a life unable to fly)...

Then the french children's illustrator told me the story about the raw meat & how he had called Toronto health about it but it took 13 whole days for them to come & remove the raw meat...Which is why the raw meat got infected with salmonella bacteria, which is why the racoons got infected with salmonella bacteria, which is why they got hit by cars, which is why I felt sorry for one & tried to take it to a emergency clinic because I didn't want to see it get smushed on the road like roadkill does, which is why I then got salmonella bacteria, which is why when 3 years later I got a Calcium oxalate lump in my breast(from Depo provera birth control calcium), which could have remained benign, but since I still had leftover salmonella Phosphorus creatures in my lungs(from inhaling them), that the lump shows Phosphate in my DIY mammograms which is why it got diagnosed as breast cancer(DCIS) which is why I am taking licorice powder & tea & eating raw vegetables & taking anti-parasitics & exercising alot alot...

Phew...Are you still with me, Jesse?

DIY Mammography: I should mention that I was taking pictures of my breast lump almost daily to track my progress...

This is how you do a home mammogram...

Take a picture with your digital camera real close to where the lump is...

Set it on Macro with Flash on always...

Upload to your computer & edit it in your edit program...

In Edit, Boost it 9 times(all the way), Move the colour slider all the way to blue, move the colour slider all the way to pink, sharpness all the way up, definition all the way, saturation all the way, contrast all the way, resolution all the way, shadows all the way... (all the way means all the way up)...

Now with the pink colour slider, start sliding slowly the other way, down a little...Watch the picture...The lump will start to appear at a certain point with more accuracy...Play with the colour sliders until you can see that lump well...

A benign lump will be almost all white(or green or whatever colour you choose-but consistent one colour)...A benign lump will also have maybe some strings of Iron...Strands...A benign lump is calcium Oxalate(oxalate means iron), those strands are iron...

A malignant lump will have some dark purple ants in it...(they may not be purple depending on what colour you choose, but they look like dark ants...) A malignant lump is made of calcium Phosphate...Phosphate means Phosphorus...

So the big difference between a safe lump & a dangerous lump is PHOSPHORUS...

Phosphorus is a component of Melanin...hence Melanoma...(skin cancer)...Melatonin is something you take to make you sleepy...Melatonin is a Phosphorus as is Valerian root which makes you sleepy too...parkinson's disease is too much Phosphorus...In the spleen...

Copper lowers Phosphorus...Licorice lowers Phosphorus because it is a copper that is easily absorbed by the body...Licorice antagonizes melanin & melanomas & skin cancers...You can apply licorice tincture topically to eradicate skin cancers...This was my big discovery in Book 3...It took me the whole book to figure this out...I say it all casually here, but it was really hard to figure out...Read Book 3 to see my journey...

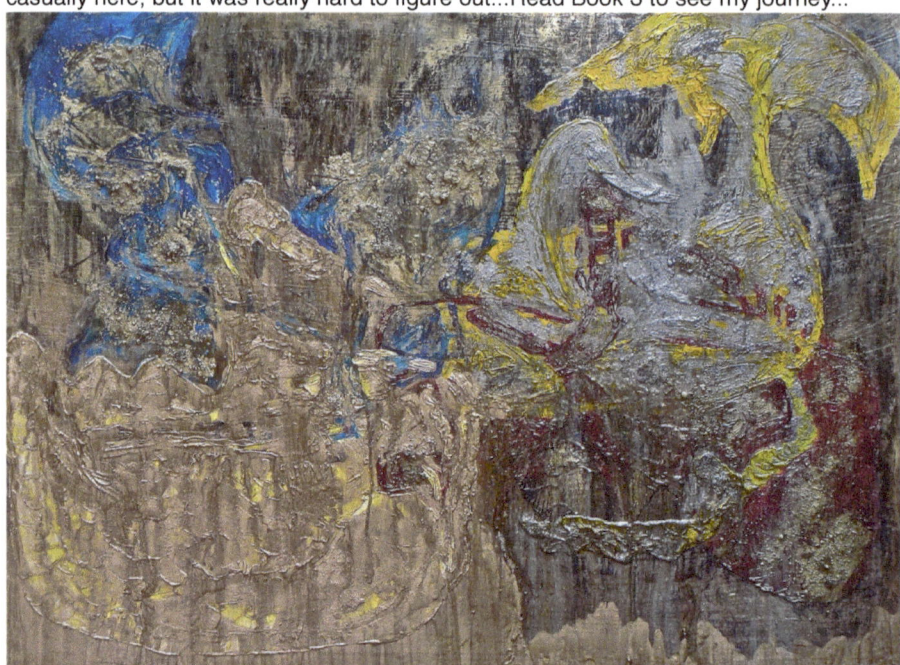

Tempesta at 3 feet by 4 feet is a walnut oil painting hand stretched with copper tacks at the sides & black carpet tacks at the back into Florida Pine wood, with tongue & groove bars(no glue)...It was stretched using a somewhat Amish technique based on temporary nails, waiting, waiting, then more permanent tacks, & a hammer...At the back it has diagonal adjustable Best corner keys which can be unscrewed or screwed to allow for temperature tension changes in humidity...Tempesta lives in the most beautiful private home of a very serious art collector...This private collector is also one of my biggest supporters as well...of course, my gorgeous, kind, mother...Don't get me wrong, this collector is not getting freebies! I am well renumerated for my troubles...The highest bidder wins & in this case it was fair & square...Tempesta was shown with Magnolia at the Agincourt Library in Scarborough which happens to be the busiest library in Toronto...(Scarborough is now part of Toronto legally)...The show was arranged by the most wonderful & sensitive Scarborough Arts organization which you should join & support because I said so...

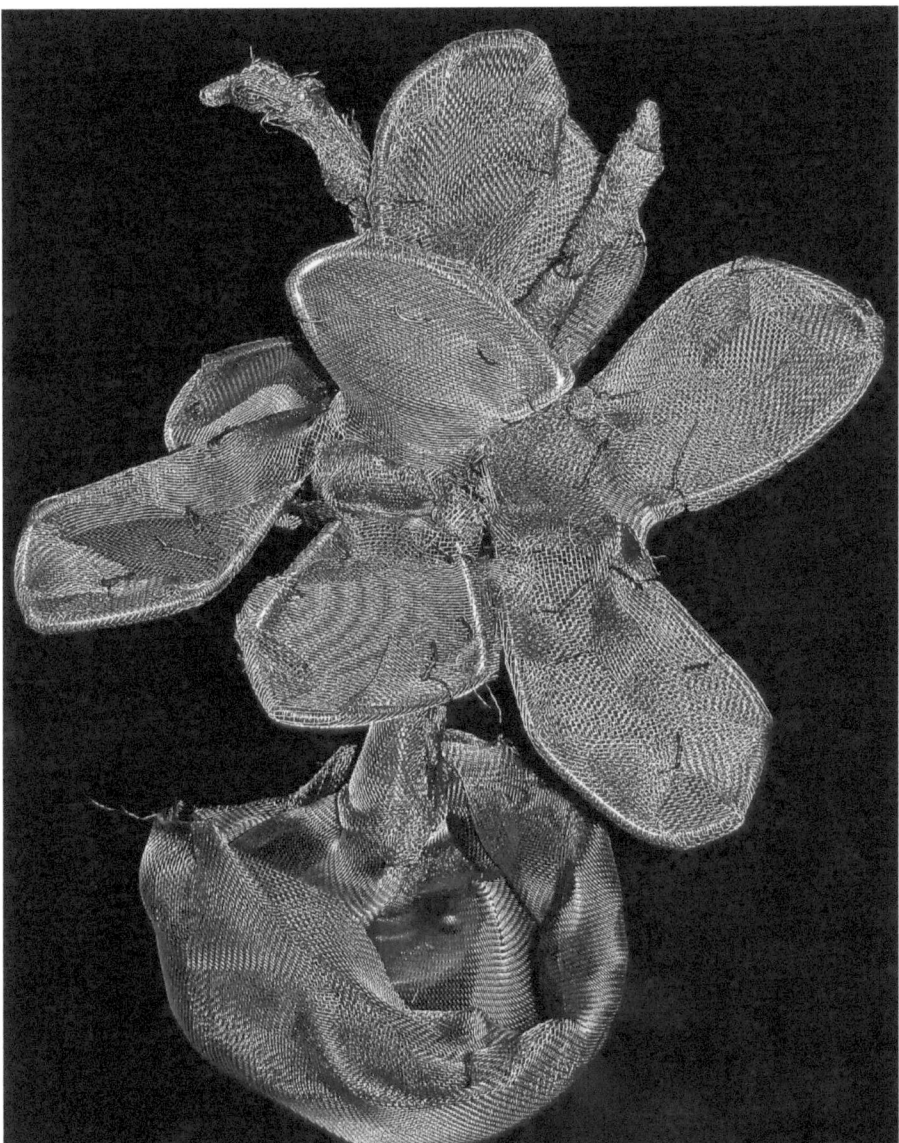

Essence of Daffodil represents Sari's breakthrough into creating a NO-WELD armature that could be strong enough to support cement, concrete, marble...This is significant because the majority of outdoor works of art in Canada are made of bronze...It is quite difficult & dangerous to weld 2 pieces of steel rod together to make a strong armature to hole say concrete on top of it...Which means that outdoor concrete sculptures are few here...With this no-weld innovation, an artist can safely build a strong underlay for concrete...This means we can have more outdoor art here in Canada, that can survive our winters here, at an affordable price, & not always in bronze...Plus there are issues with using metals from an ecological perspective...(You can see more about how the armature is made at http://www.grovecanada.ca or write to Sari Grove with questions at grove@sent.com)

Popular issues in the News on the internet lately & my opinions about that...

I think the birth control pill is dangerous...I think it causes Cancer, Gender Dysphoria & Aids...I think anyone who says otherwise is lying, ignorant or just plain wrong...I have said this before & I have explained the biochemistry in my earlier books...I also know that what they say about birth control drugs causing fertilized embryos to abort is true...I don't care much about the religion side of that, but I do think that the process will cause much weeping amongst young women who have to go through that...I think that birth control drugs are fine with many men because they don't think they have to take them...

Sadly these drugs are teratogenic, which means children are born with problems & are told they were just born that way...This saves pharmaceutical companies & so on from getting sued...Birth control drugs also cause female obesity, which is considered a leading cause of death...Despite the fact that the United States spends a huge amount on health care, it also has one of the shortest life span records in the list of countries it has been compared to...They think it is because of the very high obesity rate in the States...

I don't care if you do not agree with me...I don't think that people should be forced to prescribe these drugs to women...I don't think women should be screaming about women's rights about this...Instead of screaming, some serious person to person research should be done...You will soon learn that every woman with ovarian cysts once took a birth control drug...

You will learn that tap water in New York City is so full of birth control drugs from women peeing it out, & shoddy water treatment, that significant hormonal changes have been occurring in people who just drink alot of New York tap water straight...Did you know that fish exposed to the pee of a woman on birth control drugs have been laying eggs? Though the fish is a male fish? That study was around 2003-2004...Long time ago...

Excess Calcium in the Adrenal Gland is the actual chemical nature of a progesterone called birth control drug...if the excess is too much, the Adrenal Gland fails...hence Acquired Immune Deficiency Syndrome-yes, AIDS...The Adrenal Gland handles Immunity...When it fails, you have AIDS...Children born from mothers who took the pill, or the patch or an injection or whatever, inherit the calcium excess...if it is an extreme overload they can be born with Aids...if the excess is less than extreme, they can be born gender dysphoric...Girls feel they are boys & vice versa...

30 years after a woman was on the pill, the calcium can move down to the Spleen & cause Phosphorus excess in the Spleen...Phosphorus is like mold...Mold spreads fast...The combination of Calcium & Phosphorus is a spreading Cancer like a breast cancer...It's the Phosphorus that spreads...Even looks like a black mold when you see it on the skin...

I think women today do have the right to choose...The right to say no as well as the right to say yes...Also the right to say they won't prescribe birth control drugs...or dispense them...This is not the 1960s folks when birth control pills were considered a miracle...This is 2014 when we have tried this drug out for real...I don't like it...Read Book 3 of the Grove Health Science Series...& if you don't like what I am saying that is ok too...Dissent is healthy...We will agree to disagree...I am not going to argue the point...Write your own book if you want to say your opinion...I will not engage arguers...

"Genuine truth angers people in general because they don't know what to do with the energy
generated by a glimpse of reality." Greg W. Goodwin

(the quote above was a signature in a comment in this forum link below where people talk about salmonella poisoning(ironically it is a raw forum-yes, raw meat too...warning here btw)
http://www.rawpaleodietforum.com/health/salmonella-food-poisoning/msg44731/#msg44731

Here is a glimpse of the rough notes I send to myself by email from my iPhone using the NOTES app that comes with it...(a gold colour iPhone 4S I got used on ebay.ca & put a new battery in it using the iPHIX service guy...)

I put dashes in where something was too personal to share in a book...(names, codes etc)...

Sari's Spin on Cancer:
From:
Sari Grove <sari@fastmail.fm>
To:
grove@sent.com
Date:
Mon, 14 Jul 2014 7:40 AM (1 hour 55 minutes ago)
Show Raw Message
Show full header
Sari's Spin on Cancer:

Parasite
Hormonal
Viral

Joseph's pin #-----
Sari' pin -----

http://www.S91.ca
Goldie
647.535.----
Studio 91 hair salon

http://Artworldfineart.com

-----gore farm -----

Get licorice for copper
Hawthorn for potassium
Calcium oxalate benign
Calcium phosphate malignant
So phosphate eradication is key

Dr Jamie e-------
Mount S----

Canker melts licorice
Anti smoking patch licorice
Smithsorenson
Nicotine patch

St. John's wort tincture
Coffee 5 cups per day
Licorice tincture

Bone slow fast
Blood attaches to people like crazy
Muscle memory forgetful
Seals valves high energy
Neurons nerves renal tubes smart
Glue sugar sycophant smarmy
Water oxygen suicidal joie de vivre
Milk non sexual or sexual
Pus psychotic don't care or do care
Flesh violent mercurial Germans salt
Skin childlike adult like

Chlorine as stronger form of Oxygen
Hydrogen peroxide or hydrochloric acid as toilet descaler

Because hydrochloric acid plus Formic acid(a carbon) cleans urinals

Like hydrogen peroxide and baking soda NaC

Park I--- plumbing
Noble plumbing supply 4-- Dupont st at Bathurst

Directwaterflow P--- the plumber

http://Hidashortstories.blogspot.com

email----------------

Salmonella poisoning is phosphorus excess

Sent from my iPhone

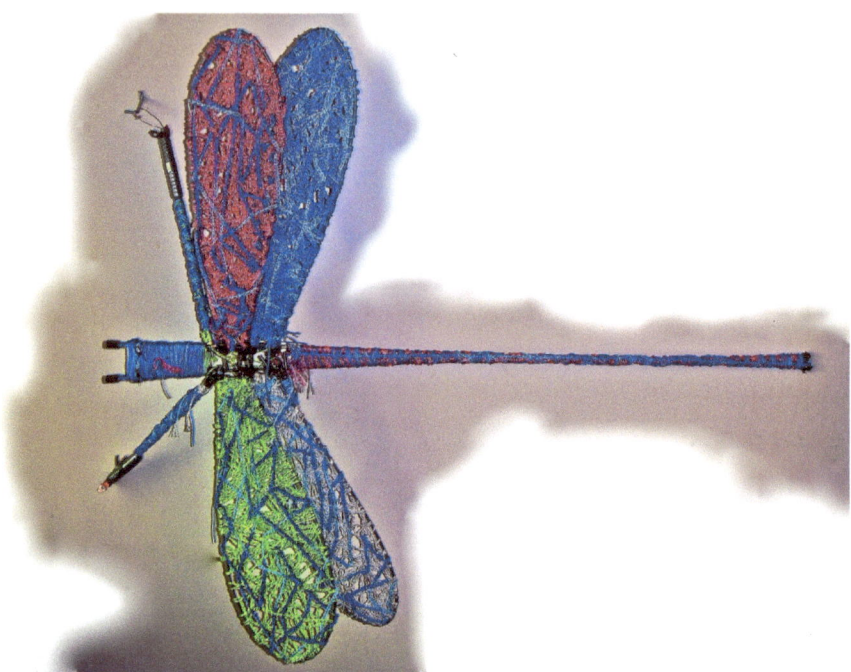

(my response to a conversation that occurred at
http://smartistcareerblog.com/2014/07/what-is-the-value-of-your-art/comment-page-1/
#comment-9711
which is the smARTIST career blog run by the most excellent creativity coach
Ariane Goodwin & the post was about What is the value of your Art?)

Ah E. ...

The pushback...

The pushback is because we as artists love giving our work away...

We love the attention...

We love the love...

I am as guilty as others...

Which is why I was seeking strength from perhaps stronger souls, maybe from the
earlier generations, but I see my mistake-older artists are not on the internet as much, I

am speaking to the already brainwashed for lack of a better word...(I mean something softer actually but cannot think of a word that I want-help me if you want)...

No it does not satisfy ALL the desires...

Just as free porn online does not satisfy ALL the desires...

A real person is better...

But porn can erode real relationships by satisfying many aspects of it, as seeing works of art online for free can satisfy many aspects...

Sorry for the analogy-it is just useful because it is so stark & brutal...

I'm not going to continue because I know you are smart...

No need to hammer down this point further...

I think you get it...

It is just a vary hard thing to correct...

We have already gone down this Alice in Wonderland pathway...

Like the musicians, it will be difficult to learn how to unshare...

We need help...

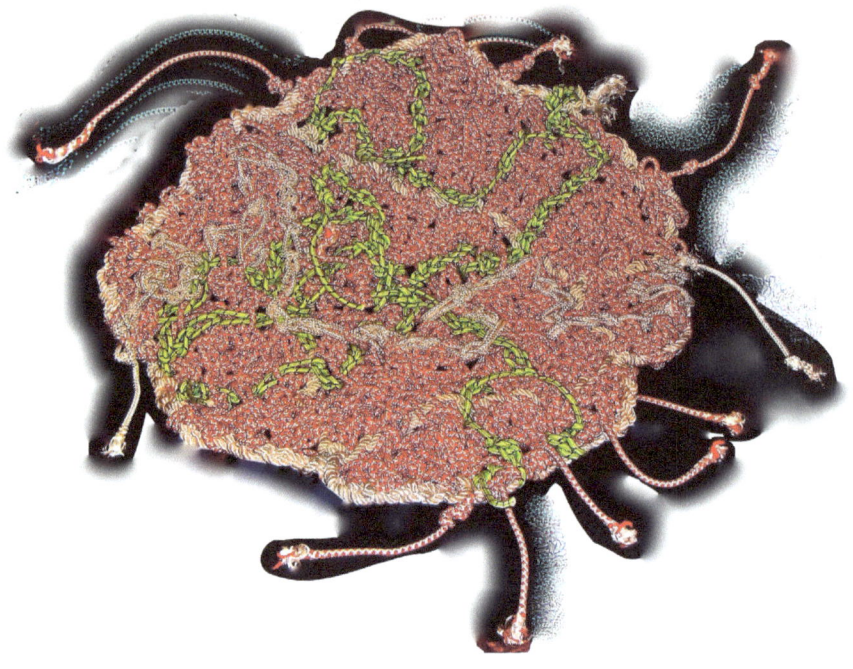

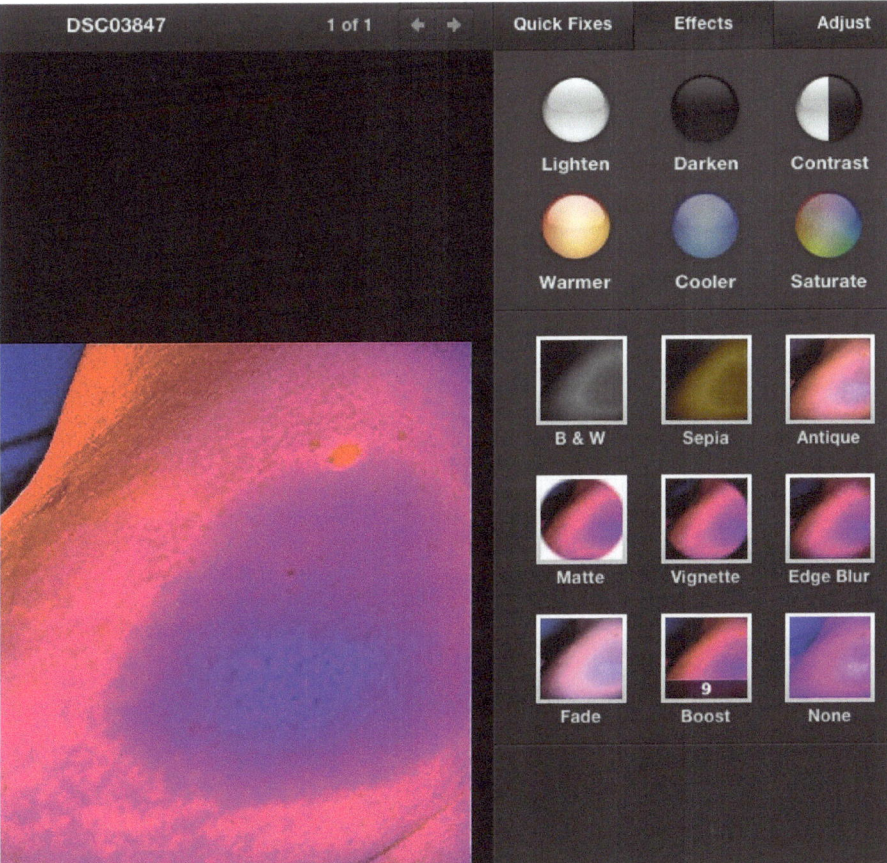

Lump 8:09 pm July 14, 2014: You will notice that the lump is significantly better than it was earlier today...The previous picture that looks like this, earlier in this book, was taken the same morning...

This picture is after a 10 kilometre walk...

I had first thing, about 4,500 mg of licorice powder(I emptied about 10 capsules of licorice root powder at 450 mg each into my morning instant coffee-with a little milk & some Splendas for taste...) I maybe ate a green apple...

I sucked on licorice root sticks while walking-purchased from The Health Shoppe at Yonge & St. Clair, East side, south of St. Clair, first block...(0.92 cents for 5 sticks)...The licorice root sticks are slightly sweet to the taste but it's not sugar...

I haven't really eaten anything all day, though at the end of my walk I had a green drink with Kale, & a few other things like Swiss Chard & lemon juice & Ginger in it which I bought at Noah's Natural Foods at Bloor & Yonge, east side, south of Bloor, first block... The picture(the above one) shows less reflectivity, which means I have lowered my iron levels from walking...iron reflects...There is less whiteness too, which means I have lowered my calcium levels too...probably from the sashimi, the sushi & the seaweed salad I had the night before...Iodine lowers calcium...All the nuts I have been eating will also have lowered my iron...

The Phosphorus ants, those purple dark spots are fewer...I screwed up with the sugar in the Poppyseed dressing-big mistake-shoulda stuck with my homemade dressing...Ruined my whole salad then I ate it anyways because I hate waste...The sugar was the big wrong there...Plus the heavy alcohol in the giant bottle of licorice root tincture & the St. John;s root tincture was a wrong...The big bottles of tinctures came with way too much booze & almost no medicine...

Joseph says that's the way with big bottles of stuff, you get less stuff, they are dilute...So I have switched to licorice root powder...Way easier to take more & the alcohol is not a factor anymore...Though I am just about to get my period & am freaking out because lumps always get worse when you have your period, this picture makes me feel hopeful this month...I am getting this thing under control instead of it controlling me...As a Virgo I like to be independent & I hate having things dictate my life for me...

Looks like things are going my way! Yay!Alot of help from strangers today...Someone said a stranger is just someone you haven't met before...Anyways, people have been nice...I guess they are reading my books & blogs & stuff & know I need some help...I'm finally start to trust my neighbourhood here & it looks like people are coming through for me...

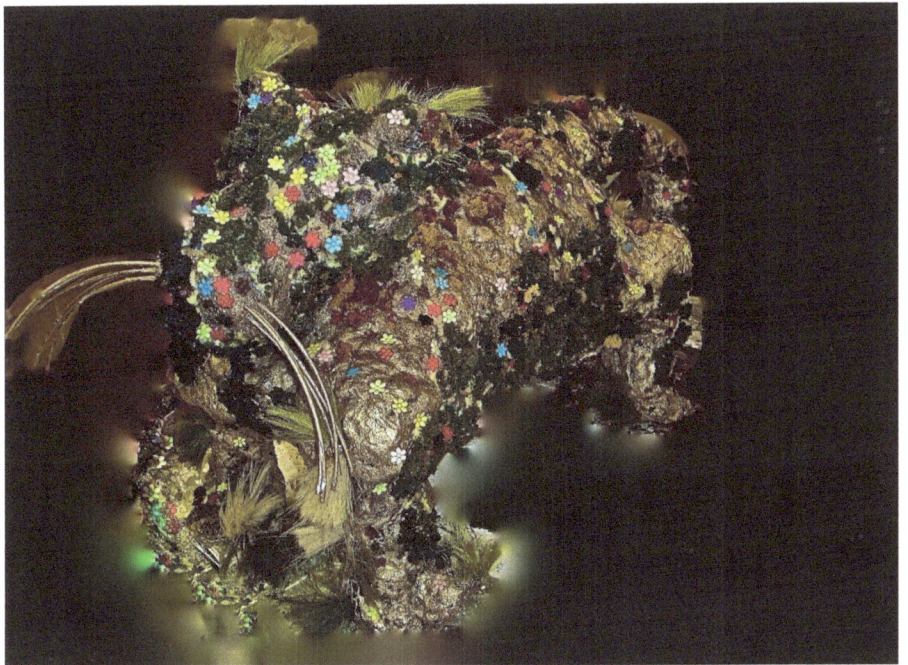

Book 5(planning-the next book is about the brain): The grove health science series

22 brain parts, paired, equals 11 body parts...

Plus or Minus are the paired brain parts...

To the Front in the BRAIN is the Minus part,

because the BACK of the Body is Female Dominant.

The left side of the Body is female dominant, So the RIGHT side of the brain is a

MINUS element (or brain Part)...

See if you can match the brain parts to the body parts?

Hint: If each CELL has 4 components, a PLus, a Minus, & a PLus, & a Minus, but

some are silent or non-dominant, & some speak which are Loud & Dominant...

Which parts are dominant in say...____---the ???

*Figure One

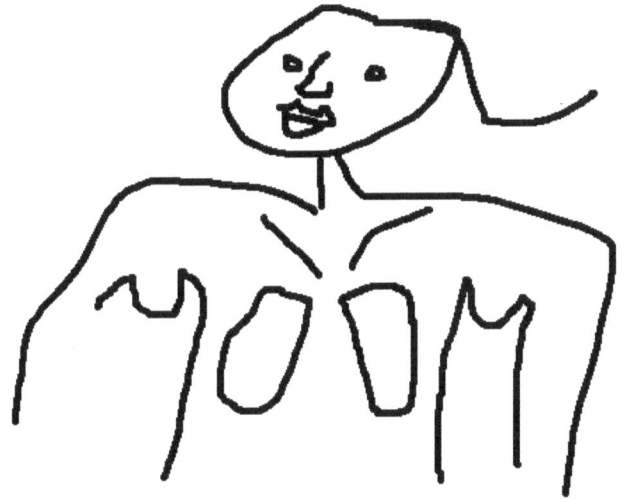

Lymph Nodes should come BEFORE Lungs on the Grove Body Part Chart...

Lymph nodes are under the armpits & provide easy access to the lungs...Spray

some Moss spray under your armpits & feel it seep into your Lung tissue in a good

way...Moss spray has Citrus Zinc, Carbon Oil, Lavender Magnesium inside! Figure

Two

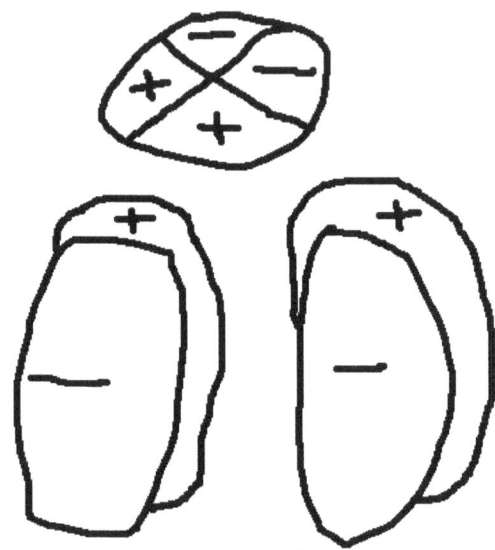

So if the front of the brain part(say in the Parietal Lobe) is a Minus female part,

& the right side of the brain part(say the parietal Lobe) is another female brain part,

Then the LEFT side of the Lung at th BACK(from the back of the person on the left

side),

is a Female body part.

Then logically the left side of the Brain part (say still the Parietal Lobe) is a Plus Male

brain part, so then the FRONT of the right lung should be a Male part (male

dominant at the Front of the Male Body Part, the Lung)...

Furthermore the rest of the brain parts & body parts should line up accordingly...

LOL!

So now we have a way to distinguish which brain parts are female dominant & which body parts are male dominant! Figure Three

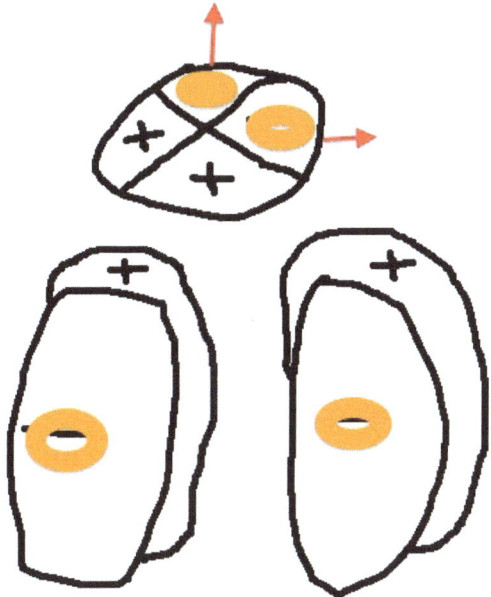

Figure Three shows a female, with, Parietal LOBE brain part dominance Minus Minus, designated by the yellow eggs, & how...

WHOOPS!!!

I am wrong I think...

If the front & right side of the Parietal Lobe is Minus Minus female, then that would

make, the Back of the left Lung Minus, & then the Left side of the Left Lung Minus,

MEANING that the Left Lung would be ENTIRELY Minus female according to the

Logic found in Book 3 of the Grove Health Science Series

"Algae+Rhythm, Algae-Rhyme:Apt Surgical Rotation App"...

Which means then that Body Parts (or Organs) would be entirely Male or female

depending on what side of the body they were on...

If logically there are 22 brain parts that pair to 11 body parts, but each body part has

 two sides, then there are logically also actually 22 body parts.

Book 4 deals mostly with curing Cancer but has some excellent things to say about

 handedness as well...

Now if everybody has two hearts, two lungs, two adrenal glands & so on, then the

Female gallbladder would be on the left side near the back, & the Male Gallbladder

would be on the right side near the front...

Which would explain why most anatomical charts

("chats" in Boston accent-joke)

 are virtually incomprehensible to

 me , a female!

Because to me, my heart is on the Left side back, whereas my husband's heart,

is on the right side front (Like he wears it on his sleeve, so. to. speak.-STS-acronym)

So if a husband is having a hemorrhagic heart event you need to apply pressure

or touch him on his Right Side Front heart level...

If his wife is having an ischemic heart event, then you need Not to touch her on her

Left side back at all...

Why? because hemorrhagic means bleeding out & missing Love, whilst, Ischemic

means Overfed & needs Less Love...

Whoops again!

The Cloves in the DIY mammogram mammography, are screw-
like...Titaniums...Attaching themselves, Antagonizing the Aluminum Winterstone cement

concrete...Figure Four

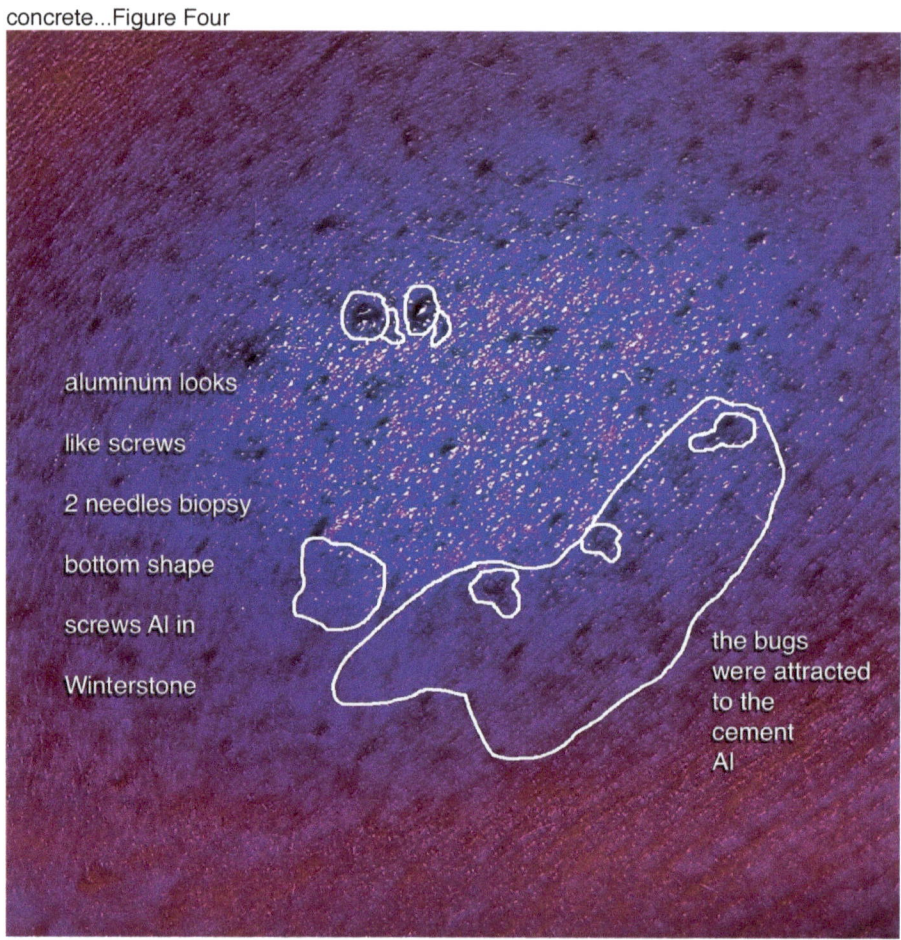

aluminum looks

like screws

2 needles biopsy

bottom shape

screws Al in

Winterstone

the bugs
were attracted
to the
cement
Al

If every mushroom cell, correction, if every cell looks like a mushroom, with a dome & a stem, or a head & a body, then the screw-like formation at the feet of the stem, at the base of the stem of the mushroom, forms when it encounters its opposite or antagonist or mate, however you want to put it...
Figure Five

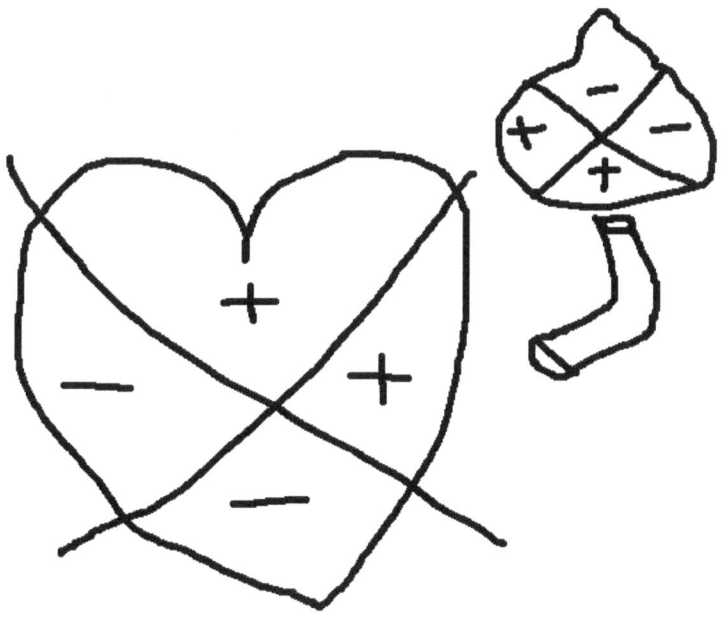

:heart: a cough is like a laugh...
Looking at the person's back side, the heart has 4 chambers...The brain, in the medulla Oblongata also has 4 chambers...
Note the positions are reversed & opposite, both...They are attached by a twisty stem inside the neck, a neural tube
(inside the Kidneys, neurons are formed, but inside the heart stems & valves are formed)...
The stem & the Valve have an opposite twist, like the Fibonacci spiral...
A twist is stronger than a straight tube...
A twisty rope, a braided twisty rope or cord or string...
If you take a clove & put it near a piece of Winterstone cement, the two will attempt to bond.
The clove forms a spiral at one end, while the head, the dome remains intact...
The Winterstone will form a crevasse, a crevice, in inverted screw-hole format...

A Valley of the Dolls so to speak-a twisty inverted valley with receptive screw shanks or threads...
A hole or black hole with inverted screw- valley in snail shape spiral but inverted...
This is how you attack a piece of cement in the lung...Cement is Al Aluminum based, Clove(the organic spice-mine from Noah's Natural Foods), chewed then swallowed, shows up in the lung picture...
Hawthorn is a Potassium based spice that can be chewed or made into a tea or powdered(grinded)(grated) & eaten swallowed drunk.
Hawthorn attacks or mates with Aurum Gold like Taurine powder or rabbits.
Hawthorn should be found in celery or celeriac the root of the celery stalk.
Saint John's Wort is the top of the Anise plant & is a gum cleaning Copper like in Diet Coca-Cola but weaker & safer...
Essential oils can be put into carbonated water, oxygenated water, to make a bubbly soft drink...
Alcohol is just water, Hydrogen, but when it sits for a while it gets heavier, so, more Hydrogen. (so like H or H2 or like H3 or like H4).
H4 will attract more Oxygens, like 2 of them, because H2O is water, so maybe 4 Hs gets 2 Oxygens.
So Hydrogen PerOxide is like baking soda plus vinegar which is a Zinc.
So Carbon(baking soda plus salt) + Zinc (Vinegar) equals an Oxygen.
Salt is NaCl, which means salt + a chlorine which is Oxygen.
So chlorinated water is Hydrogen with Oxygen with Salt which is a lesser form of Mercury Hg & Silicon is somewhere in between, but all in the Mercury category on the Grove Body Part Chart.

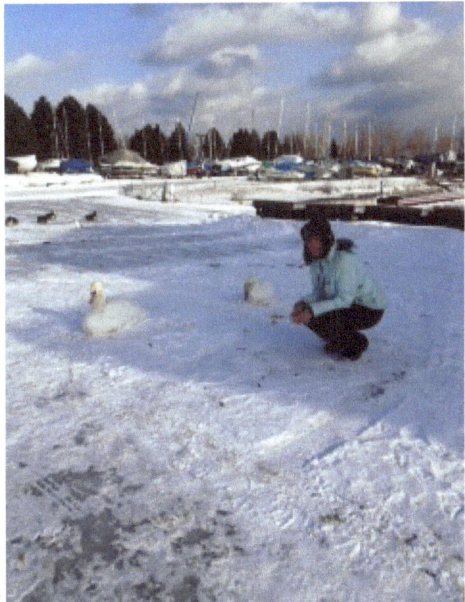

Figure Six:

Fighting is like sex... For example: Raccoons sound like they are fighting when they are having sex...Screaming & shrieking...But is sex like fighting? When you have sex are you really actually just fighting? Hurting each other on purpose? Then stop...Stop having sex if you are just actually fighting...

Figure Seven

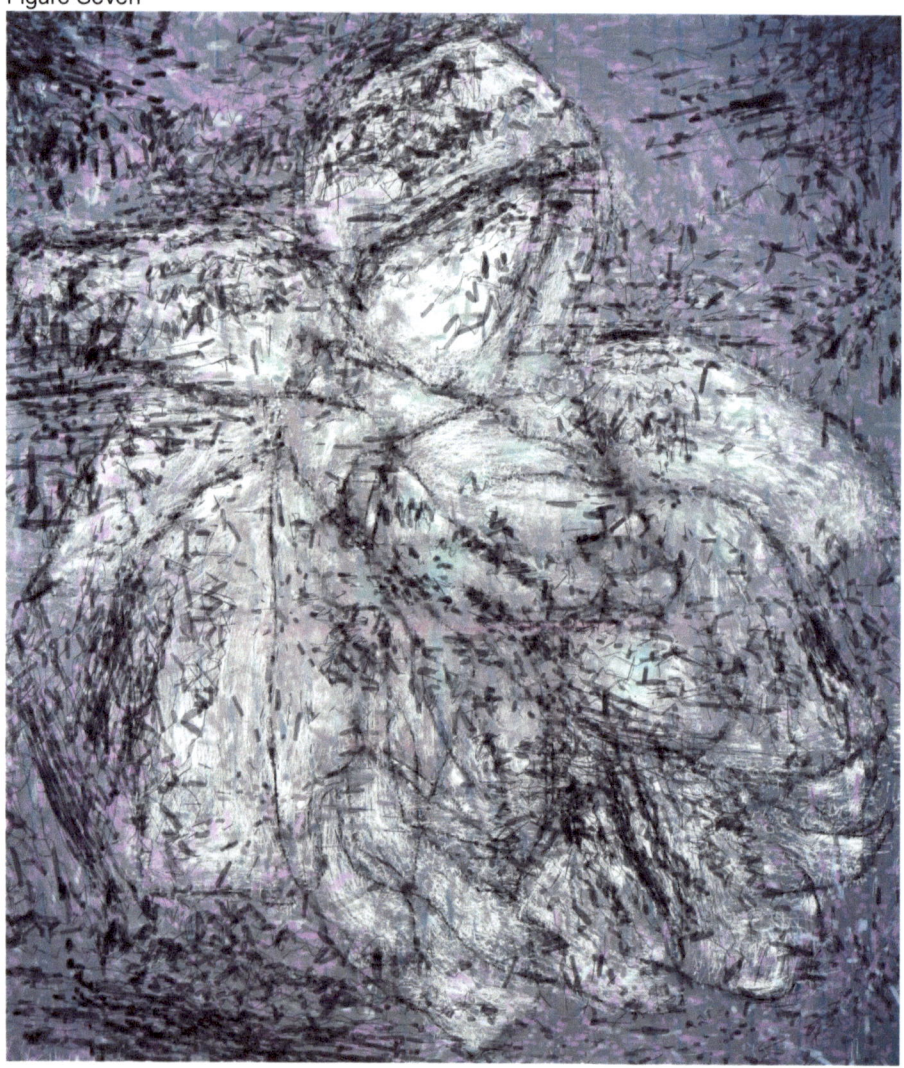

Figure 7; Kale contains both Iron & Nitrogen...A "bowl of Kale" might be pronounced "Bolakale" in Nigerian, maybe? People in Niger speak French & are maybe good with pottery, clay & bowl-making?

*Ebola is just a Nitrogen excess in the Kidneys, treat with a Carbon like an oil...Trees distribute carbon well when they are alive...Sit under a tree...Vegetables contain Nitrogen, so back off the vegetables a bit, & the leafs, the leaves...
   *Carbon, from Carbon type generators can be ignited to make heat using fire or flame...If you don't use enough fire or flame then you distribute an excess of carbon, oil...This will make you stupider...

*If you distribute sufficient fire or flame to burn off Carbon but not pollute with Excess Carbon, then you can have fire bound/generated heat, that makes you warm, WITHOUT electrical outlet needed or even electricity...

There are devices today that will do this safely...

A wood burning fire makes heat as well in the winter months, which can be called November to April in Toronto...(Six Months)

Figure Eight:(Blender 3d animation still photo png)Unedited iPhone 4S Notes follow, by co-author. S.G. 2014

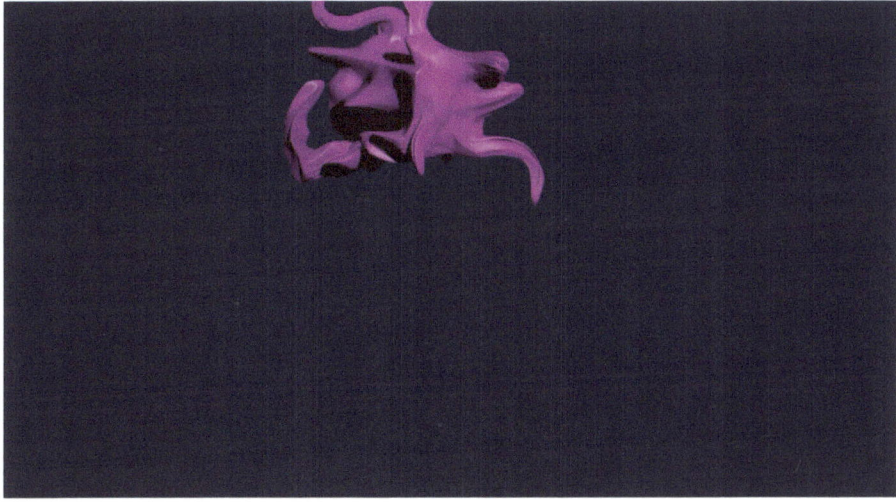

Crazy due to oxygen air condition units periodic cleaning hydrochloric acid bleach ingest zinc vinegar baking soda carbon salt = oxygen chlorine
Symptom heat rash legs

Das tut Mir leid

That blows my light

Car washes gasoline phosphates from cemetery into water supply of Greenhouse juice company

Rainbow trout eats turquoise is between flesh and skin Arizona stone soft phosphorus phosphates

Coffee licorice root folds teeth Montreal good Je me souviens

Medulla oblongata at back of neck shape of an X
Front & right gap of X are Minus
Left & Back gaps of X are Plus
In brain
In body the Heart with shape X
Superimposed
The left & back of heart are Minus female
Right & front chambers Male
We are seeing the whole picture from
Behind
& slightly above
This is our perspective of the Heart...

Screws-Aluminum forms screw shapes in cement...
Winter stone is white with screw shapes metal pieces screws Aluminum ground in...
You can see them...
Very tiny screws...

Correction:clove cloves form screws when encountering mate Aluminum Winterstone...
All cells are mushroom shaped, like head is dome.
Stem is body.
Forms screw at base of stem when it encounters antagonist white boat upside down of Winterstone cement!

Brain power
 turtle barracuda
 hair

Haiku
Farm

Ebola is high Nitrogen

West Nile is malaria is high sulphur in Pancreas treat with Tonic Water quinine garlic antibiotics insulin

Eat fish Sari

Black walnut leaf tea Mn
Licorice root powder Cu
Vega one sugar free energizer Zn powder w/ ginger 'n turmeric Zn
Water hot boiled H

Anchovy oil wavy blue capsules
Emptied out my kidneys well
Especially the left kidney

Phosphorus came from a strip club hence the cocaine...

Drinking bleach as a medical procedure? Baking soda + vinegar= bleach or NaCl C +
Zn H2O = O4(hydrogen peroxide ice cube adds freon)

Spare the rod spoil the child
Rape is violence
Violence is the rod
#RCChurch

Doctor forms to fill out

Give someone enough cocaine they will crave the Phosphorus

5 stages of death
Birth, person, couple, person, death

Sent from my iPhone

Figure Nine:

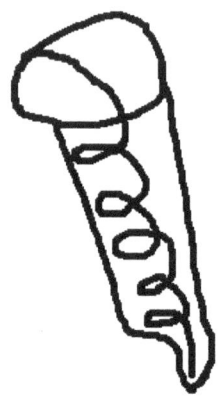

Pancake Corn Grit Oil fried might ameliorate recipe if corn grits too "dry" ie:Nitrogenic...

Nitrogen Laundry (causes Ebola? if clothing is Calcium cotton based causing clog in Adrenal Gland blocking for a while, up to Kidneys...)

Cloves attack Aluminum in cement or concrete or Winterstone
Fig. 9 shows how Clove spice chewed then swallowed with liquid ends up in Lymph Nodes first, then into Lungs, mostly left lung tissue, but some in right(left for ladies, right for men),

then forms a screw shape as it meets an Aluminum object...like cement...or cocoa beans from chocolate...Figure 10: ibid

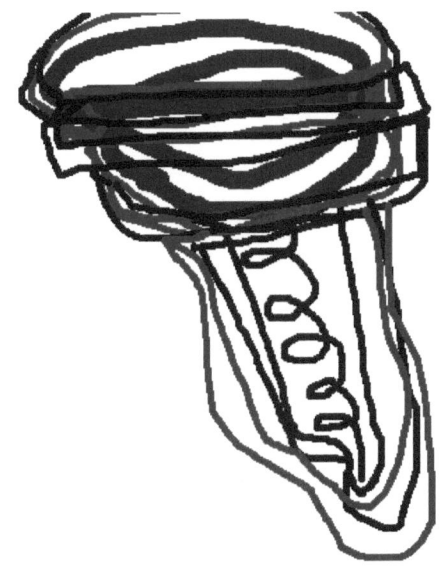

Fig. 10 shows a leaded screw, a galvanized screw has ZINC Zn on top, hot water strips Zinc from pipes, lead pipes that once were galvanized, & makes them just Lead pipes, then lead goes into water & ice cube water...

Lemon juice

(squeeze half a lemon & drink juice-seeds can be eaten for Oxygen or spat out for not)

 worked to dissolve Lead
Plom Pb component of concrete, the metal part, like a cockroach is mostly Lead...

Lead

Bleach is Baking soda sodium bicarbonate Carbon plus Salt C + NaCl(chlorine is just an Oxygen but more)

Zinc is Ammonium or Ammonia or ACV Apple Cider Vinegar

equals= Oxygen

So Bleach is 2 things added together to make Oxygen...

Basically $Zn+C=O$ for simplicity sake

You could die from drinking bleach...

Oxygen

In the "Flow" feng Shui of things, the Lymph Nodes actually get fed BEFORE the Lungs...NOT after...

Lymphs

Fig. 11

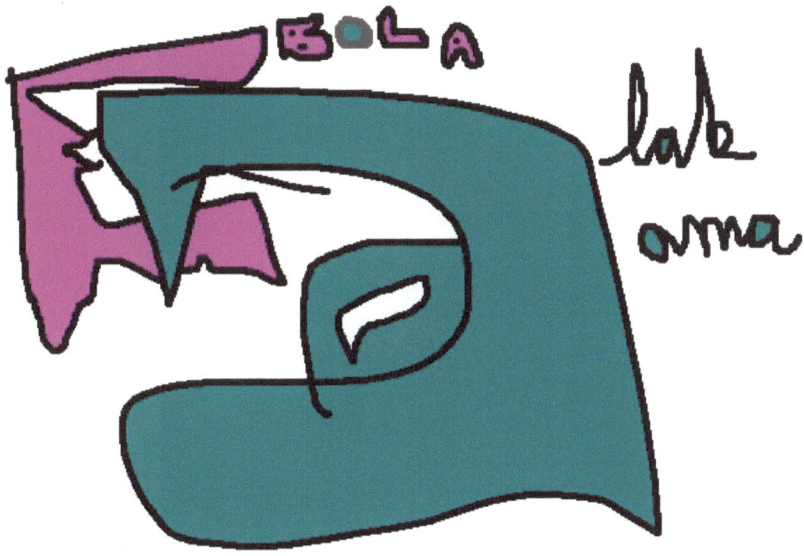

Figure 11 is a mention of Ebola which is a Nitrogen excess in the Kidneys...Treat with Carbon, any oil, food grade, meaning edible...(drink half a teaspoon of olive oil with half a teaspoon of squeezed lemon juice every morning)...

Blisters are wetness...Because when you sweat, Hydrogen in your sweat is thing. like it has substance, so it creates more friction than if your feet were dry...Water has weight, & size & mass, making your in essence bigger than before when they were dry...A dry foot is a smaller size than a wet foot...Blisters are caused by friction...Dry your feet often when walking far, & bring a change of socks for mid-day changing of socks...

Lymph nodes first then lungs...The armpits are where the Lymph Nodes live, & they precede the Lungs & the Breast tissue...A perfect way to clean out the Lymphs & Lungs is to apply stuff to the armpits...Rub your medicines into your armpits to clean out your Lymph Nodes & Lungs & Breast tissues...

p.s.Did you know that a Needle Biopsy is actually 2 puncture wounds into the area where your Lungs are? This causes lack of pressure in the Lungs & can cause trouble breathing...Vitamin A can patch those wounds but Vitamin A can also exacerbate the hardness of a lump-ie: makes lumps harder...So after a needle biopsy, take 2 weeks off work to let those holes heal up so you can breathe again...

Strip Clubs carry a whole mess of airborne dangers...Fluorine gas & liquid fluorine in the water supply & air...Cocaine fume in the air as well...Phosphorus is in the air too from the excess male & female ejaculate...Phosphorus is what makes a tumour malignant, so just breathing in the air at a strip club can cause tumour malignancies...Don't believe me? This is why the strippers are fed a constant diet of cocaine...Because the Copper in the cocaine can offset Phosphorus ejaculate...But it is a careful dance, dangerous, to tempt fate in this way...Freon gas from air conditioning is constant as well...Freon, Fluorine & other anaesthetics are date rape drugs...Which is why so many men get raped in strip club bars & taverns...

Lithium lead bonemeal olanzapine zyprexa...Are all in the Vitamin A carrot & potato family...

You gotta let the water run for awhile...After your water has been shut off...You gotta let the water run for a while or you will be drinking your neighbour's sewage water...

.....................................ll\ (B'elanna typed this)...Bengal cats have maybe a 400 word possible vocabulary...As do many animals...Teach your family friend words...Animals can speak as well as write, paint, talk, & listen...Some speak foreign languages too...

scooby
scoby
system of accepting/finding fault in others
mushroom kombucha/choade nitrogen
ferments down to p phos. smell

Mushrooms, which are Nitrogen dominant foods, can be fermented...This creates a breakdown of nutrients...So you get Nitrogen, Sulphur, Hydrogen, Calcium, & Phosphorus...This is beneficial if you have over-medicated against parasites & are in need of healthy bacteria...Or if you have drunk bleach...Or something else stupid & dangerous...SCOBY is an acronym for that list of bacterium...It is just food, don't be afraid...Over-washing, people who over-wash, may also need SCOBY...You can get it in probiotics, fermented cabbage products like sauerkraut, yogurt, & this new trendy thing called Kombucha which is just fermented mushroom sometimes in black tea...

licorice root powder on cats worked!Cu. against P.

Sprinkle a little licorice root powder on your cats if you think they have a Phosphorus parasite...Licorice root powder is a Copper like catnip...This is how cats clean themselves in the wild-they chew catnip...In India Neem...Anise...In Somalia "Chatte"...

st.John's Wort is a form of Cu. cleans gums. Diet coke.

noix de muscade.
mugwort. nutmeg.

Mugwort powder lowers iron in the Blood, in the Thymus gland area...Iron makes a lump reflective...In photography...See Book 3 of Grove Health Science Series for info about how our DIY Mammography techniques were developed...

unscoby.
Se. O.Io.Cu.
carbon.selenium.oxygen.iodine.copper

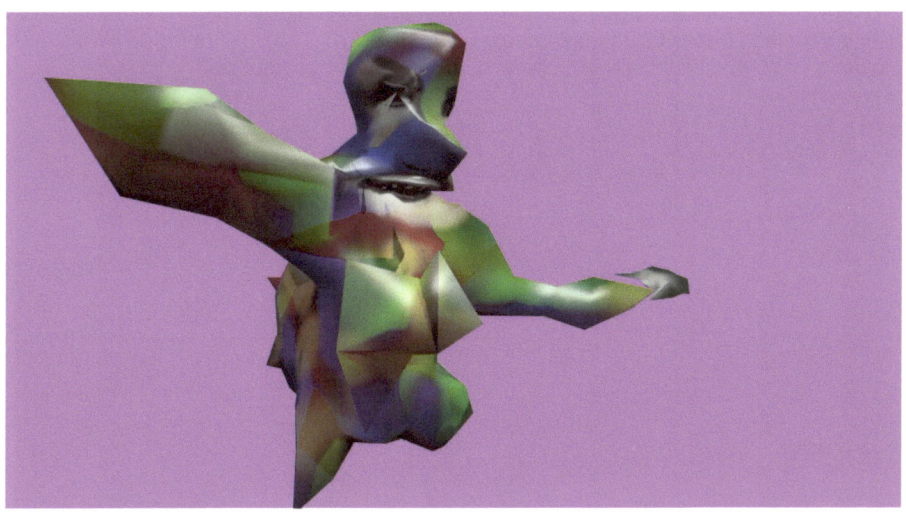

bbbhhhhhhhhhhhhhhh

a cough is a laugh

the violet, the top of the violet plant, the flower, contains iodine...re:#madagascarperiwinkle

Vega One Sugar Free Energizer Powder contains Ginger & Turmeric which are both in the ZINC family...If you take any anti-psychotic drugs which are based on Lithium, Lead, Bonemeal, or Vitamin A, like Potatoes or Carrots, you should know that those anti-psychotic things will cause a breast lump to grow...They make breast lumps harder, the lead Plomb in french language...Zinc things remove Lead Plomb PB on the Periodic Table of Elements...

On Blindness, Cataracts etc:

Usually a Sulphur excess in the Pancreas...Think sugar when I say Sulphur...Too much Sugar is the most common cause of blindness & is of course associated with Diabetes...

Now, I know of someone whose husband took her to a Transylvania type eating club where they served fried chicken blood...After that, this person, whose eyesight is legally blind, showed some slight improvement in seeing ability...I am guessing the iron from the fried chicken blood was the source of the improvement...

I also know of someone who had lost their sense of taste & smell, for several years, & was given a blood transfusion, & both senses came back...Again, I am guessing the Iron from the blood was the source of the regaining of abilities...

Possibly, a diet change away from Sugar & towards iron might help with blindness & seeing troubles...I see many people cheating themselves of healthy iron filled meals by snacking on sugars...Perhaps this cheat is the source of eye troubles?

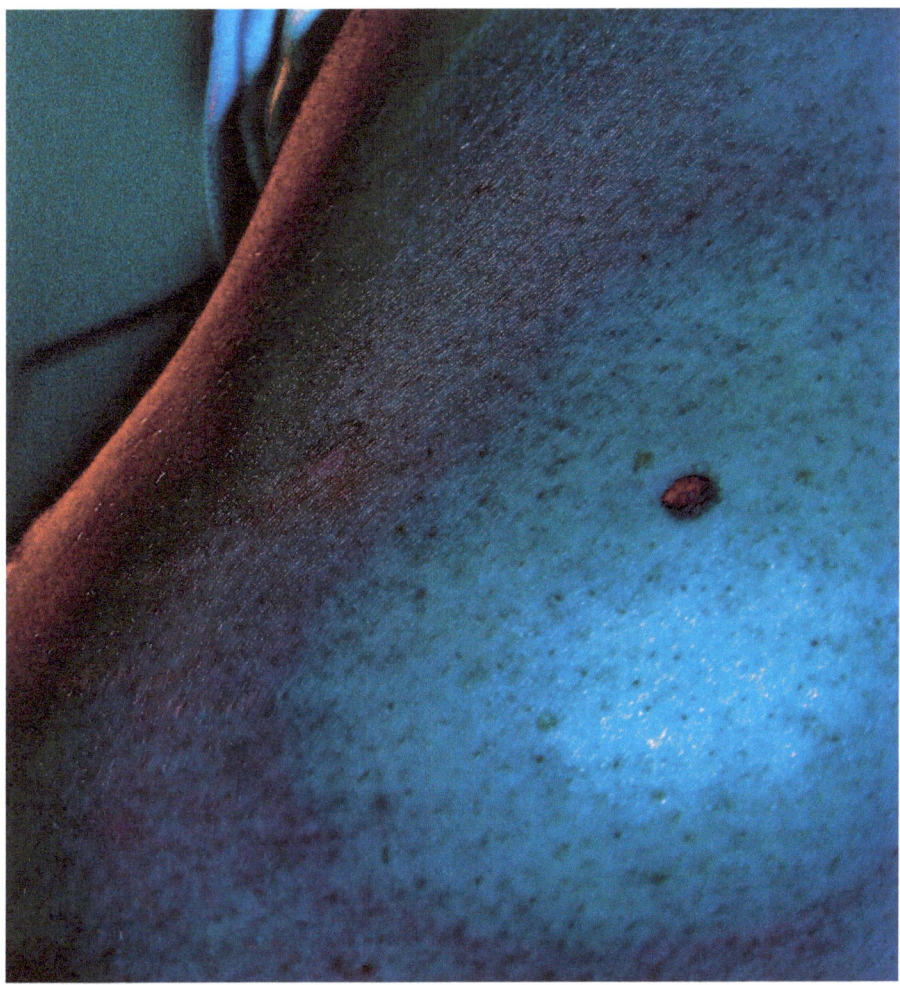

Saturday August 2nd, 2014 at 8:31 pm...

Notes on eradicating a breast Cancer lump:

1)Track the lump by photographing it with your digital camera set to Macro with Flash On...Upload to your computer...
In EDIT mode, Enhance...Boost all the way...Boost definition, sharpness, resolution, shadows, all the way...Slide the Colour bar ALL the way to Blue...

Slide the other colour bar all the way to Pink...
Slowly slide the Pink slider down a bit & stop when you can really see the Lump well & what is in it...
Those purple ants are Phosphorus & indicate malignancy...

You want to get rid of ALL purple ants to get rid of breast cancer!! So make LICORICE ROOT POWDER part of your daily medicine diet-just stick like 4 tablespoons of it into your morning coffee!
The white blob is calcium...

Iodine things eradicate Calcium...Chew Madagascar periwinkle for Iodine, or Poke root powder or Poke root tincture, or Iodoral tablets, or eat seaweed salad or fish or sushi...
The reflective nature of the white is IRON...

Iron makes the lump hard...Manganese things lower iron, so eat Nuts which have manganese...
Mugwort powder is a manganese, goes fine in tea...Nutmeg is a manganese...Lead or Lithium or anti-psychotic drugs or bonemeal or bone or meat or potatoes or carrots all contain LEAD the element & that will make the Lump BIGGER...

ZINC things remove lead...I like vega One sugar free energizer powder with Ginger & Turmeric cause they are both Zincs...I also love VITAMIN D3 drops for the Zinc...Very powerful in liquid form the Vitamin D3...

Have ordered Vitamin D3 in 50,000IU as capsules...This is because I am getting impatient to get rid of this lump fast...Am getting huge pressure from family members to cave...

Am eating mostly raw diet now, for example:

Salad of green apples, tomatoes, Apple Cider Vinegar, Olive Oil, Mustard with Horseradish, walnuts, various seeds & dried cranberries, sesame seeds, broccoli, kale, cabbage slaw, avocados...& so on...

I have found that meat makes the lump bigger & worse...I have found that cooked food, even vegetarian cooked food does NOT give me enough energy-RAW vegetarian food does...

Cheating with fish or seafood seems fine, especially Vietnamese & japanese cooking like Sushi or Pho...(Pho is Vietnamese broth with raw stuff you toss in like lemongrass leaves or bean sprouts or fresh Mint leafs...You can ask for vegan broth Pho...Ossington & Dundas Pho restaurant in Toronto, is large portions & cheap prices & awesome PHO!))

Continue one day walk 10 kilometres, one day rest schedule...

Go to sleep very very early, wake up feeling happier with the sun...
Netflix helps for when I am too tired to move after the 10 km walks but not able to sleep yet...

Diet Coke, Diet pepsi, Diet GingerAle, excellent!

Licorice Root powder is most important ingredient to eradicate the malignant nature of lump, the Phosphorus...DO NOT FORGET THIS!!!

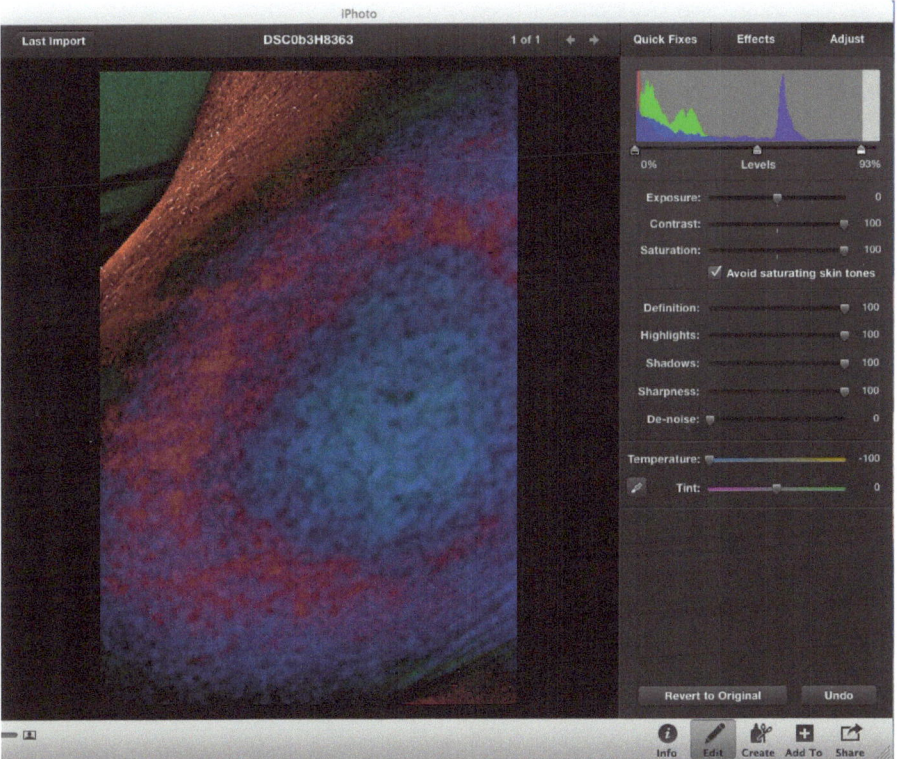

DIY Mammogram made easier...

by GroveCanada

So you found a lump in your breast...You are freaked out...You immediately go raw vegan, walk 10 kilometres a day, drink wheatgrass & licorice root powder & take high potency Vitamin D3 capsules...Awesome...(BTW-these are all things that I am doing & DO recommend)...

But how do you know if all this is working? How do you know if things are getting better? Well, start taking pictures...You may not know this but your point & shoot digital camera can see under the skin to your lump...With your computer's editing program you can even see the chemistry of the thing...

This is a photo of a lump in my left breast...Taken with an 8 megapixel Sony DSC-T100 point & shoot camera, set on Macro, with Flash on, held just a few inches from where the lump is, in the bright light of my kitchen...

Uploaded to my Mac desktop snow leopard, to the iPhoto program...Go to Edit...

First, ENHANCE...(in Quick Fixes)

Then in EFFECTS, click on BOOST as far as it will go(9 times for me)

Then in Adjust, see the setting in the picture below...

I have Definition, Highlights, Shadows & Sharpness ALL the WAY Up...

Most importantly I have BLUE ALL the WAY to BLUEST...

Saturation all the way up, Contrast all the way up, & I have checked avoid saturating skin tones...

There you go...That's it! You can now see what your lump looks like...

The White is Calcium...To get rid of calcium you need Iodines...

Reflectivity is iron...To get rid of iron you need Manganese...

Purples are Phosphorus...Phosphorus is what makes these lumps spread...To get rid of Phosphorus, which is the MOST important thing to get rid of, you need Coppers...

Copper is found in Licorice root, Wheatgrass, St. John's Wort...So my favorite thing for turning a malignant lump into a benign lump is Licorice root...Alot...

Every day you can take your own picture & see how your lump is doing...Fewer purple ants? great! That means less Phosphorus & less Cancer!!!

This will help you to track your own progress as you try to get rid of your lump...

Sometimes the medicines you take will make things better...Sometimes worse...This is a great way to check...

Sari's Protocol right now for getting rid of a breast cancer lump:

Walk 10 km a day...

Eat only raw vegetables (but cheat with fish or seafood to get some protein)

Take licorice root solid extract, tea & tincture daily(licorice is a Copper that antagonizes Phosphorus, Phosphorus is the thing that makes a lump malignant & scary-licorice root has been shown to cause Phenotypic reversion, which means it turns a cancer cell back into a normal cell...

Take Vitamin D3 50,000 IU(yes it's alot) once a week(Vitamin D3 antagonized Lead which is what makes a lump big...This is an important one to take plus it gives you tons of energy)...

Take Manganese daily(like 4 x 25 mg pills)(Most lumps are calcium Oxalate which means calcium & iron...Manganese(NOT Magnesium) directly antagonizes Iron so taking MANGANESE will eat away at the iron component of a lump)...

Note:Sari has already taken so much Iodine that she cannot take anymore or it will push her into early menopause-HOWEVER, IODINE is crucial to an anti-cancer protocol if you haven't taken it before...You can get Iodine in Iodoral pills, kelp pills, Madagascar Periwinkle herb, Vinpocetine or Vincristine supplements, as well as seaweed salad, sushi, sashimi, fish, seafood & various other things like Arame a sea vegetable you can cook...

Oil-Olive Oil as salad dressing, with Apple Cider Vinegar, & Mustard with horseradish...These 3 items are a great salad dressing combo...

Sari's daily salad includes:cabbage, nuts, dried cranberries, pumpkin seeds, walnuts, green apples, avocados, cherry tomatoes, various sprouts & sprouted beans, sesame seeds, love...

Have added 3 Junior chewable ibuprofen tablets after my Welsh friend sent me a study about aspirin eradicating cancer cells...

Coconut Water hydrates very well & is a total laxative...(for after your giant walks)...

Netflix-this is my reward for after my long walks...Eat a giant salad & watch Netflix...You will be too tired to do much else...

Walking Notes: If it is warm I wear Teva hiking waterproof sandals...
Long shorts with many side pockets so you can carry stuff & you look normal if you decide after your walk to go grocery shopping or something...
Tops with built in padded bra so you don't look all flattened out like most shelf bras do...
Halle Headbands on Etsy provides my awesome headbands-looking awesome is important...
Thong underwear means stuff doesn't ride up your butt-well, I guess it already is, but I find thong underwear more breathable & less annoying or rubbing during long walks...
MUSIC- ROCK MY RUN! It's an excellent music APP for your iPhone that has terrific playlists you can just play with no download...Get an arm strap holder thing for your iphone too-mine straps just above my elbow...

***Walking 10 kilometeres(about 6 miles) a day is a FULL TIME JOB...But having a lump in your breast is dangerous, so I think the walking is more important than anything else...You will be too tired to do much of anything else, but at least you will have a sideways chance of getting rid of your lump...Without the exercise you are not in the game...

Additions:
Have added Wheatgrass powder(another Copper)...Dissolves nicely in black tea in the morning for some extra energy...
Have also added Black Cumin supplement capsules...(also a Copper like Licorice)

So what is a breast cancer lump made of? (& how to get rid of it!)

August 15, 2014Painting Edit

A benign lump is made of calcium Oxalate...Oxalate means iron... So a regular lump is Calcium plus Iron...

A malignant lump is Calcium Phosphate...Phosphate means Phosphorus...Like mold...Phosphorus is mold & that is why the thing may start to spread...

So...

If you have read our book "Grove Body Part Chart:A Medical Arts Innovation"(see our website to read it free online or buy a paperback), you will know that COPPER antagonizes Phosphorus…So to stop a lump from being malignant, you need a Copper…

I use Licorice root…Licorice root solid extract is a syrup that is highly concentrated…Licorice root tincture is the extract in alcohol…Licorice root tea is good too…You can chew licorice root sticks…You can get licorice root powder…Licorice is a highly absorbable Copper so it really hits the Phosphorus in your body fast…

Ok, so now you have changed your lump from malignant to benign…

How will you know that your licorice root regimen has worked & the lump is indeed free of Phosphorus?

Check out the previous post to this one for my DIY Mammogram instructions…

Basically you take a picture close-up with flash on in Macro setting, of your lump…

Upload to computer, then in the EDIT program(like iPhoto) do these steps…

Enhance in quick fixes, then in Effects Boost it 9 times(like all the way you can), then go the ADJUST area & go all the way up for-Definition, Resolution, Shadows, & Sharpness…Most important slide BLUE all the way to BLUEST…

You will now see your lump close-up…Take a picture before taking the Licorice root tincture, then at the end of the day(give at least 2-3 hours after) take another picture…This might be too fast, but if you are lucky you will see the difference right away…

Your first picture will show a white shiny lump with some dark purple "ants" in it…The ants are Phosphorus…

The second picture should show fewer ants…

A benign lump is almost all just white & shiny…

A malignant lump has dark purple spots or ants in it…

The licorice root however you take it will eradicate the purple ants, removing the Phosphorus & making your lump benign…

Ok…   You

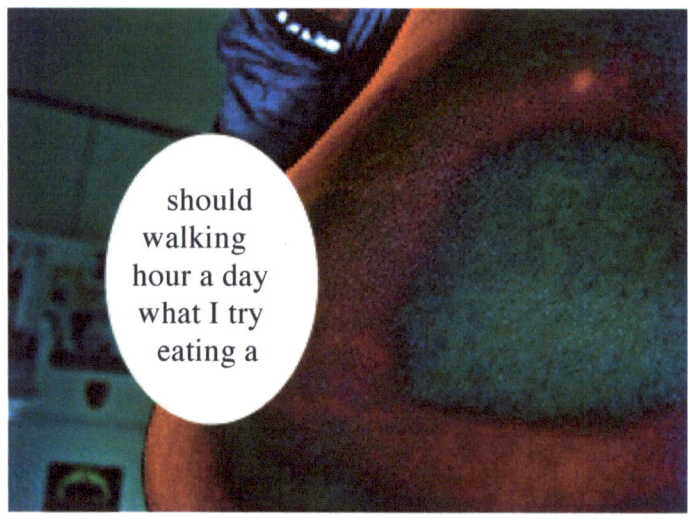

that | should | know
an | walking | over
km is | hour a day | (10
& | what I try | for),
| eating a |

mostly RAW vegetable diet(I cheat with fish & seafood) will make the whole cure process faster…

But now…You still have a lump…benign, but it is still there, bothering you…

Ok…What you are left with is the Calcium Oxalate(Iron thing)…

Iron makes the lump hard & your body has trouble reabsorbing it…

If you read our second book "Do it Yourself Medicine:A Repair Manual" (see Sari Grove's profile on the Independent Author's network to see all 3 published books in the Grove Health Science series),

you will know that MANGANESE Mn (NOT magnesium Mg which is totally totally different) dissolves Iron…

Manganese dissolves iron…

So to soften up the hard exterior of your now benign lump you need Manganese…

I've just been taking Manganese supplements…More than the recommended dosage by the way…Play that by ear…You need enough to make the lump softer, but not so much you get sick…

I should mention that the big anti-Cancer thing going around right now is called "Bloodroot"& is a Manganese…Opium is Manganese too…Nuts & sesame seeds are Manganese…I put a large large serving of sesame seeds into my salads…Poppy seeds are Manganese…Mn is its acronym on the Periodic Table of Elements…

The problem with Bloodroot is it is so strong it makes you sick & vomity & just well sick…Too strong & very dangerous…

The Bloodroot salve is dangerous too…The theory is correct, but taking this thing is, well, dangerous…

Bloodroot tincture, dissolved in water, can be taken orally, very dilute…You could try that…

But I am sticking with plain old Manganese supplements(just little powdery pills you can get anywhere easily), for safety reasons…

Ok, so now you have made the lump softer…

All you have left is calcium…

Our 3rd book "Algae+Rhythm, Algae-Rhyme:Apt surgical Rotation App" explains my whole weird journey in figuring out all of this… (you can get free tiny Kindle versions on Smashwords of our books-smaller than the pay for Kindle books on Amazon, but still eminently readable)!

So in our 3rd book you learn that IODINE antagonizes calcium…

A great very absorbable supplement that is in the Iodine family is called VINPOCETINE…

It absorbs better than the Iodine pills…You could also just chew & swallow the herb called Madagascar Periwinkle to get Vinpocetine…This is a cheap & very effective way to go…Just eat the herb itself…

But if you are lazy you can buy Vinpocetine supplements which are derived from the madagascar periwinkle herb(called Vinca Minor) …This will dissolve the calcium…

There!

This is my recipe for how to get rid of a breast cancer lump!

I'm Sari Grove…

p.s.The whole process of everything in your body happening goes way faster with a ZINC…It speeds up all everything…Vitamin D3 is a ZINC…I have VitaminD3 capsules which you can take once a week & are 50,000 IU…Awesome…Don't take too many or you will go bipolar…Really…

p.p.s. Make walking far your job…Every day if you can…6 miles or 10 km….It is a full time job…

p.p.p.s. Eat only a raw vegetable diet & cheat with fish or seafood for protein…This will significantly improve your chances of success…Raw vegetables give tons of energy…Cooked vegetables not so much…If you do a cooked vegetable diet you may feel dizzy or lack of energy or just hungry all the time…The raw diet will mean you don't go hungry…I lost 25 lbs right away…

Lastly…Get some Hawaiian Coconut oil & get a good suntan…The Zinc from the sun helps stuff to move along, digest, reabsorb…The oil is good for you too…Drink Coconut Water to hydrate & as a laxative…Poohing alot is crucial too…

Hugs…Sari

Hello,

My mum asked me to send you some info about what I am doing-basically a non-surgical regimen(includes walking 10 km daily & a raw plant based diet), but more importantly, what chemistry I have been taking to dissolve the thing using biotherapy & epigenetics…
Thank you for your support!
I am doing very very well, happy that I have nailed this protocol down finally!!!
(Book 3 explains the journey including false paths…Book 4 explains the solutions that worked)…All are free reads online at http://www.grovecanada.ca
Sari Grove(Carol Slatt's daughter)(also daughter of Dr. Bernard Slatt-neuro-ophthalmological surgeon)

 Subject: DIY Mammography & Sari's progress at eradicating the thing NON-surgically…Breakthroughs!

Date: Fri, 15 Aug 2014 18:41:36 -0400

Hello, (re: the idea of taking the picture with a measuring tape in the photo)

So the measuring tape pictures came out not exactly…

I hold the camera so close it made the measuring tape seem like the lump was 2 inches…

But it is not even one inch…

I don't have metric on my measuring tape…

I decided a while ago that nobody understands metric most of the time…

Anyways I sent you an earlier photo…

The white is Calcium...

The shiny is Iron...

The dark spots(which are now very few) are the Phosphorus, the hormone receptive stuff that is like mold...

The "antidotes"(antagonists) I am taking for each element of the lump are:

For the Calcium I take an Iodine-Vinpocetine is a great pill for Iodine...(You can also just eat the herb called Madagascar periwinkle for the Vinpocetine, which I also have at home & is cheap & easy to get, it is a good tea too or boil it & drink...)

For the Iron I take Manganese...A basic manganese pill...(pills actually)

For the Phosphorus I take a Copper...I use Licorice root tincture...

Every day sometimes 3 times a day I take a picture & edit it for colour to show the chemistry of the lump...

Getting rid of the dark purple spots was the first priority...(Licorice root does that well)

Next was reducing size...(Manganese does that well)

Last will be forcing my body to reabsorb the Calcium via the Vinpocetine(Iodine on the periodic table of elements)

I track all this in my books which can be read for free at
http://www.grovecanada.ca

Book 3 tells of my journey to how to solve this lump problem...

Book 4 tells my solutions & is there to read but is being updated all the time...

Sari Grove

p.s.feel free to forward this email to whomever you please...I have cropped the photo for modesty & the information here is so good people should be privy to it...Plus the books need to be read, this is a good teaser! (LOL)

Note:The red dot in the picture is a scar-nothing to do with the lump)
Attachments

Morning update(Aug 16, 2014)

here is this morning's picture!

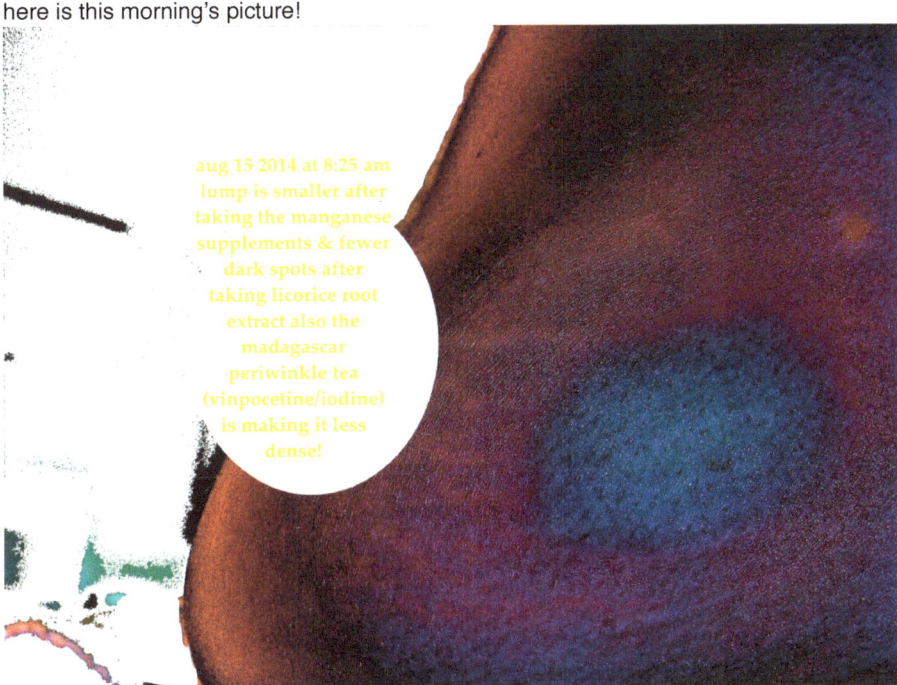

aug 15 2014 at 8:25 am
lump is smaller after
taking the manganese
supplements & fewer
dark spots after
taking licorice root
extract also the
madagascar
periwinkle tea
(vinpocetine/iodine)
is making it less
dense!

smaller! yay!

making progress with the manganese pills, licorice root extract syrup,
madagascar periwinkle tea protocool…

***(Mn, Cu, Io…these are the symbols for those 3 elements on the periodic table)

****(They antagonize these 3 things- Fe, P, Ca)

am going to look for a measurement ruler for pictures program now to
help me measure inside pictures…

Ok…(Later this morning of the 16th…9:57 am)

Turns out measuring things in Macro in a picture is hard to do…

So this is what I did…

I took out my measuring tape & guesstimated how big the lump is by feeling it…

About One inch exactly today…

So that means that in the picture, the circle of the lump is about one inch in diameter in the photo…

So, in the free Mac Paintbrush program, I drew the circle & put some rectangles beside it with notch marks just to help me guide how big things were in Macro…Note:My notches are not real measures, I just needed something graphlike to get an idea of how big things were by eyeballing the notches & the circle…

Here is that hand drawn Macro Ruler…

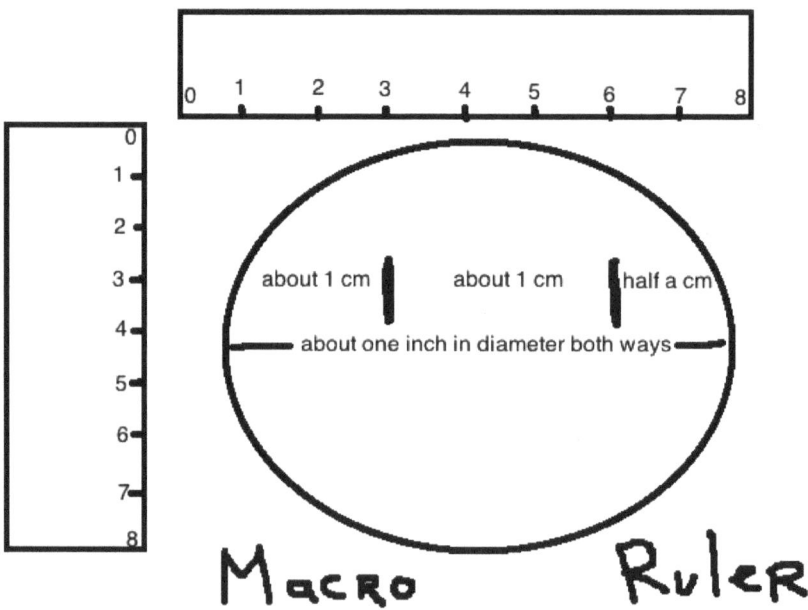

So again: The circle in the picture is the same size as the circle of the lump in my Macro real picture of the lump…

Ok so then…

I opened the real picture of the lump in Mac Preview…

Then I opened the picture of my new Macro ruler, grabbed the circle in the ruler picture, & pasted it on top of the real lump…

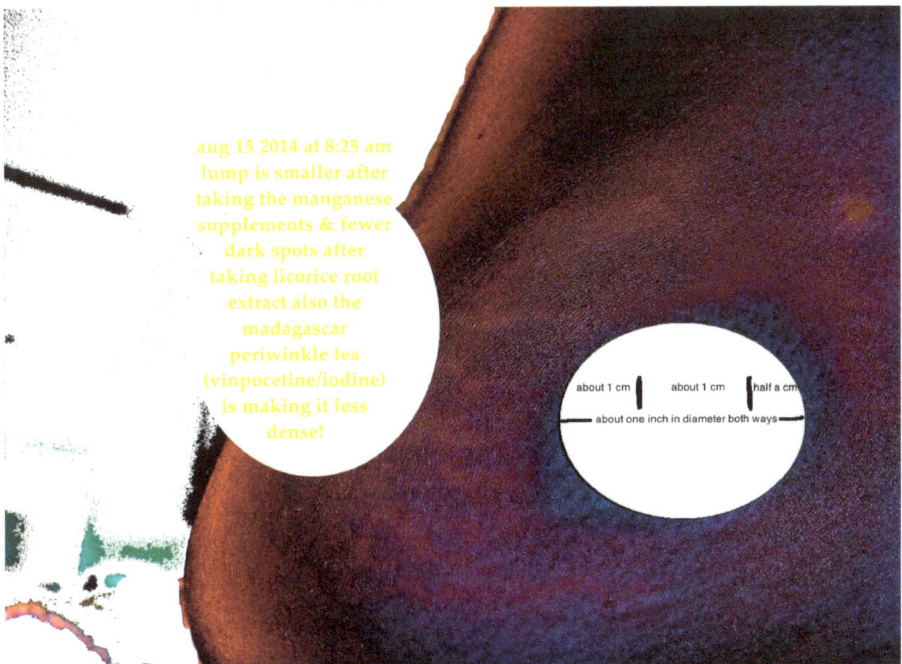

aug 15 2014 at 8:25 am lump is smaller after taking the manganese supplements & fewer dark spots after taking licorice root extract also the madagascar periwinkle tea (vinpocetine/iodine) is making it less dense!

about 1 cm   about 1 cm   half a cm

about one inch in diameter both ways

Of course, the circle sits on top of the lump easily because that is my control circle…

But tomorrow & the next day & the next, I can use this same control circle, just pasting it on whatever new Macro picture I take…

This will help to document in pictures, how the lump is shrinking with my protocol…

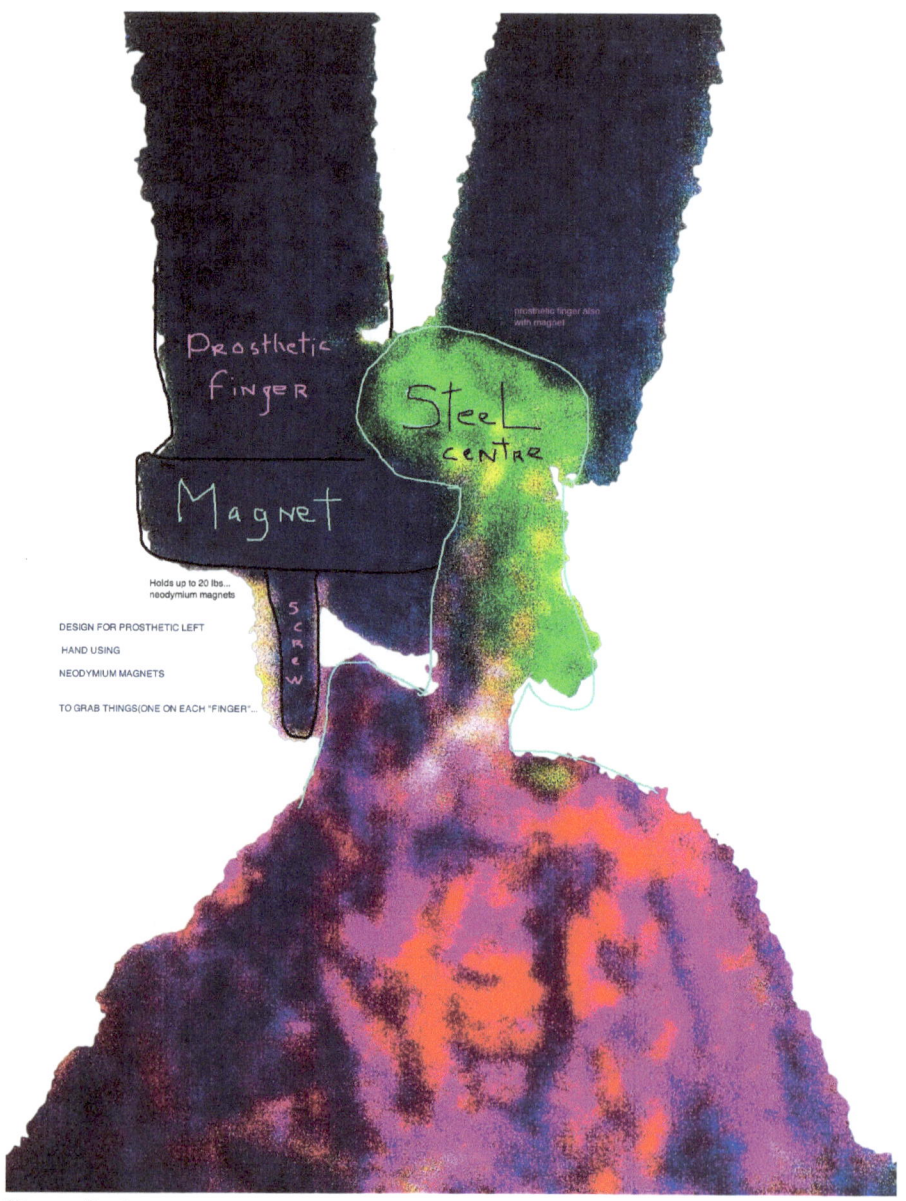

Theory Engineer...

The link between salmonella bacterium & cancer(& Pneumonia) & how to solve the cancer problem & how I went from theory to engineering solutions...by Sari Grove

How I got to where I got:

I knew that the raccoon that I tried to rescue had eaten spoiled raw meat...

I knew that I had contracted some sort of bacterium...

I knew that raw meat when it spoils attracts salmonella typhi infection bacterium...

I knew a Cancerous lump was made of Calcium Phosphorus & a benign lump was calcium Oxalate...

So I knew the differential between benign & malignant was the Phosphate, the Phosphorus...

I was able to see pictures close-up of a calcium Phosphate breast lump...

I was able to see close-up what Phosphate/Phosphorus looks like...

On a hunch, I went to see what Salmonella looks like close-up, guessing that if the raccoon, & then I, had both gotten Salmonella, that my new breast cancer lump was somehow related to salmonella bacterium...

I was able to see a picture of the salmonella bacterium close-up... Simply put, the picture of the Phosphorus in the Calcium Phosphate Cancerous lump, & the picture close-up of the Salmonella bacterium looked alike...

As an artist I am skilled at seeing things, similarities & differences...

Again...If you just look at the Phosphorus component of a cancerous lump, it looks like purple ants in the picture...In fact, better pictures show the ants truer in colour as a turquoise colour...Phosphorus as a rock mineral is turquoise...

Take a look at a salmonella bacterium up close...Turquoise ants...Same shape as the weird dark spots in your lump...

It even shows up when you take your own Macro photograph of your own lump using the DIY Mammogram editing tips I outlined in "Grove Health ScienceSeries:Book 4"(about $15 dollars right now on Amazon as a paperback)...

So that is how I made the correlation between a breast cancer lump & the salmonella bacterium...

Also:I know Copper antagonizes Phosphorus...I know licorice root is a copper...So taking licorice root tincture should eradicate the Phosphorus/Salmonella from my breast lump in pictures...& it did...

Once you eradicate Phosphorus from a breast lump it is no longer a Calcium Phosphate lump...It is now just a benign lump made of Calcium Oxalate, Oxalate means iron...

Manganese dissolves Iron...Take Manganese pills (easy to get are 25 mg pills & I take just way more than the recommended dosage to get an effect-maximum maybe off label dosage to dissolve lump might be 10 pills x 3 times a day, stop if you feel vomity),

to dissolve the iron nature of the lump...

Iodine dissolves Calcium...A good herbal plant called Madagascar Periwinkle can be boiled & drunk as a tea & that tea contains Vinpocetine which is a highly absorbable form of Iodine...

(You can also buy Vinpocetine pills for more money & not necessarily better results)...
(Madagascar Periwinkle is also called Vinca Minor)... Eat a raw vegetable diet...
Cheat with fish or seafood because they are high in Iodine...
Walk 10 kilometeres a day(6 miles)...Cheat by sleeping some days when you are tired...
Bread, breaded coatings, cereals, crusts, grains, glutens, can make the lump larger &
block up your digestive system, cause bloating, & generally slow down your nonsurgical
breast lump removal program...
Sugar doesn't help either...
Artificial sweeteners like Stevia or Splenda contain one sugar molecule & 4 potassium
molecules...Potassium actually lowers blood pressure so these are fine...The one sugar/
sulphur molecule shouldn't worry you...So these are all fine...(though if you have Low
blood pressure be careful with art. sweeteners-they will lower it more)...
Water & Alcohol contain Hydrogen...Hydrogen makes lumps bigger...So cancel that 8
glasses of water a day idea when trying to shrink a lump...Water makes lumps bigger
actually...Same goes for alcohol...
(Now alcohols can contain other things which may be good for shrinking a breast lump
& if you are thirsty water is good for you there...But this whole drink lots of water thing is
not correct when you are trying to shrink a lump...Water is a food...Think of it that way...)
If you are fasting, but drinking liquids, liquids act as your food...In those cases you do
need to drink because you are not getting any other nutrition...
If you are a salt eater you can carry 15 lbs of water in your system from just water
retention caused by the salt...This will make your lump bigger...Cut out salt...This will
help you to lose that water weight...
Sari Grove Sunday, August 17, 2014 1:39 pm in the afternoon Toronto, Ontario, Canada
with Joseph Grove's help.../ & the cats... B'Elanna Grove:intact female silver bengal cat
b. Dec. 1, 2004 Jadzia Grove:intact female gold bengal cat b. April 16, 2005

Mad cow disease is like Lyme disease, a mercury excess in the gallbladder...
(citation:Book 2 Grove Health Science Series)<DIY medicine:A Repair manual

Kuru is the theory that if you eat an older person's brain that it will dominate your brain
sort of...That the older person's brain is dominant at the point of fresh eating, so you
should wait until it biodegrades before eating it...Hence the theory of cemetaries & burial
system , whereby the brain spoils & degrades down the Grove Body Part Chart list(from
top to bottom-Book 1)...Meaning: Like Kombuchu, which is Nitrogen mushroom tree
heart

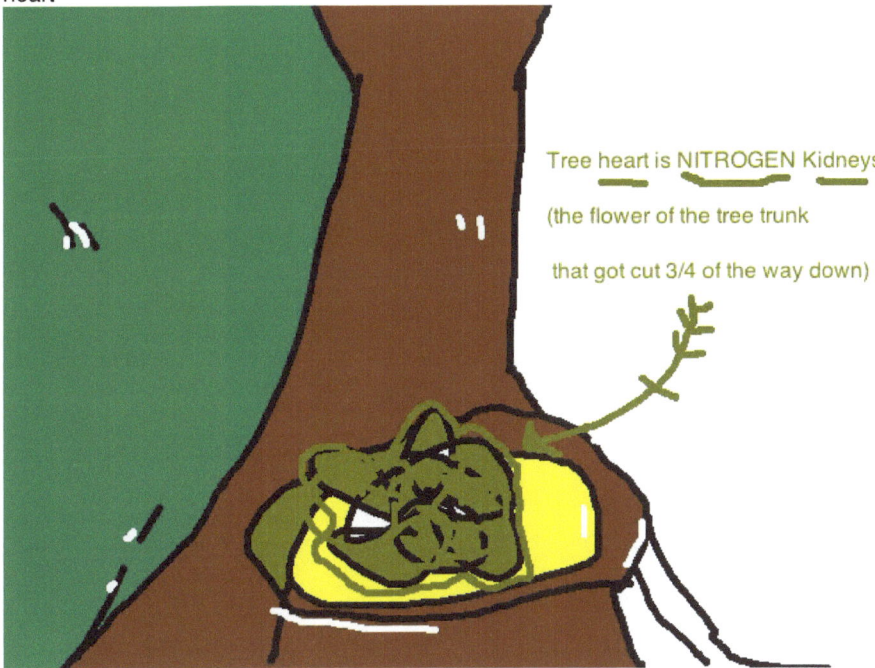

Tree heart is NITROGEN Kidneys

(the flower of the tree trunk

that got cut 3/4 of the way down)

'

what I mean to say is,

The Tree in the picture Tree heart, has had the front trunk cut down 3/4 of the way
down...

The Nitrogen heart flower sprung up...

The true colour was a yellow green mushroomy colour with beigey accents which is a mushroomy colour...Mushrooms are a NITROGEN element...

A tree has a mushroom heart that flowers internally like a floret, in scalloping scallops...

Trees have mushroom hearts...

So back to the point: Kombuchu is Nitrogen mushroom fermented (by waiting) down to its composite parts, all the way down to a Phosphorus...

ie:

Nitrogen Kidneys Plus element,
Pancreas Sulphur Plus element,
Hydrogen Liver Plus,
Adrenals Plus Calcium,
Phosphorus Plus Spleen...

Add some Black tea (Cu Copper Minus spleen) & you have now convinced somebody that probiotics (think like yogurt) are good for an anti-cancer protocol)...

They are not...

Probiotics are the opposite...Probiotics are fermented things like mold which promote mold like Cancer...

Black tea is a Copper which kills mold...

Hiding yogurt or mushrooms in black tea is a SNEAK...

A sneak is a sneak...

It also might mean someone is trying to kill you with probiotics by making you moldy then you die a slow horrible death of mold infestion & oozing Nitrogen gross mushroom-like ooze like the BLOB (from the film The Blob)...

Or they are trying to patch up that hole(2 holes actually) in your lung from the needle biopsy which is causing you to feel like you cannot breathe & your lungs keep filling up with fluid when you try to drink cold water...

Or they are eclectic iconoclastic idiots who are tree hugging Druids who want you to figure things out on your own because you are a pain in the donkey...!

So remember that in Homeopathy- opposites attract ie: for example, if they say the sky is blue it is red or pink, if they say eat yogurt then drink black tea, if they say drink black tea eat yogurt & so on...Homeopaths can be very Sneaky people...

Naturopaths might be safer...ISIS at Yonge & St. Clair... is a Goddess...

Next topic for re-consideration:

Ballon catheters are just a tube with another tube inside with a balloon stuck on the end of the inner tube but not blow up...You stick the first tube into the person...Then you stick the inner tube through the first tube...Then you blow into the inner tube & the balloon on the end swells up fills up...Then you can push a spine back into alignment...Acupuncturists do this with electro-acupuncture needles & it is usually safer if it is done by someone who really is Chinese from China & was certified there & maybe doesn't even speak English that well or not at all but knows what he is doing...

A nurse is not the same thing as a doctor...I repeat...A nurse is not the same thing as a doctor...

A student nurse is not the same as...

A person who graduated high school & wants to be a nurse is not the same thing as a Head nurse who might have a PHD in nursing...

An accident is an accident an accidents happen & that is called an accident...

In Canada we brought in No Fault Insurance which means we understand that both people or neither people might be responsible for an accident-we usually call that Acts Of God...There is a section of the New testament called "Acts" which is about Acts of the Apostles, which is about stuff they did & some of it was acts of God maybe & some of it was acts of the Devil maybe & some of it the Dragon & some of it the Beast & some of it we just don't know how they did what they all did...(Georgia peach accent)

Bless your Heart!

A beetle is a shiny bug...Beetles come in boys & girl genders...No need for a microscope...

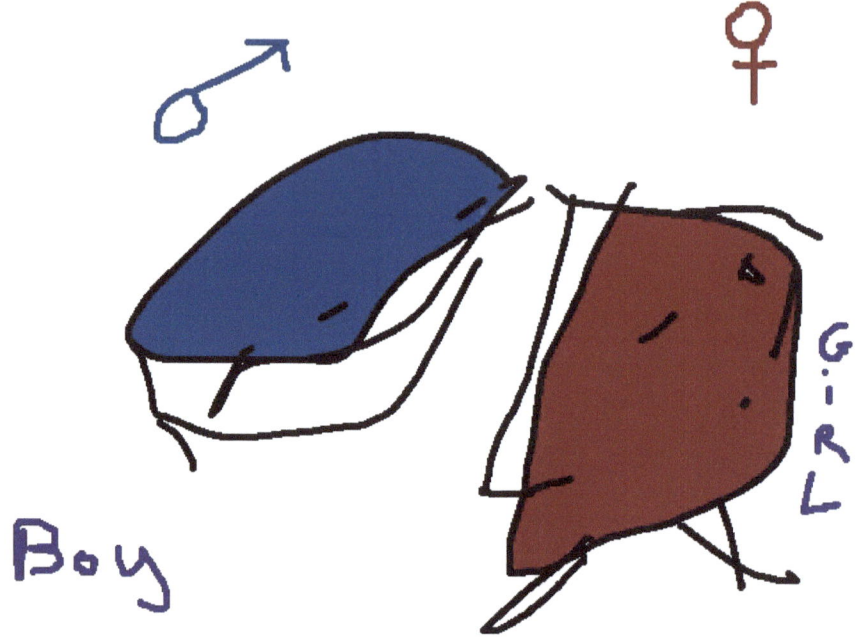

Generally speaking in Nature the boy will be behind the girl but on top (if they are humping) lol smile...

Other positions are outlined in the Kama Sutra but that is yoga & not my field...The Hare krishna Temple has yoga & also free soup & funky haircuts...But you may have to wear sheets as clothing & tamp on a tambourine t airports to protest airplanes & wear flower lays in your hair...(Hawaii flowers maybe, a Lua? pronounced LU-OW)...

Decibel Levels...

Above 80 is illegal Even between the hours of 9-5...

40 is allowable between 9-5 but is annoying to neighbours...

20 is normal for traffic but can be dangerous if extended into sleeping hours ie: nightime

10 is reasonable between couples fighting...

Water or proximity to a lake increases sound due to echo...
Silence is Golden...

Signs is a restaurant for hearing impaired waitstaff...Sign language & reading lips is understood...

There is another restaurant Black & White for visually impaired waitstaff...It is in the dark...

The World Trade centre cement & concrete made its way to Canada in the form of recycled cement...

St. Marys is the cement company who know how to recycle cement, who knows how to put white Portland cement into smaller bags that won't break your back, & who knows that Baby Powder the magnesium type (not the cornstarch type) can help to dissolve cement lung gently if applied topically...*A more interesting method of dissolving cement in the lung is through the use of Cloves the Spice(organic)...You can even see those cloves attacking, drilling into the cement like fusilli if you take a picture of your lung using your own digital camera set to Macro then editing as I described earlier in the DIY Mammogram instructionals...Clove powder can be found in capsule form at the Gingko store under Holt renfrew at Bloor & Bay in Toronto...Empty the capsules into a liquid & drink-it may numb your mouth a bit...

St. John's Wort is the top part of the licorice root plant...Anise...It makes your gums tingle like cocaine does but is an herbal form so LESS...St Johns wort is a COPPER which is good for cleaning out your mouth area...The TOP of a plant the green parts is usually better for the top part of your body ie the brain...The bottom part of a plant like licorice ROOT is usually better for the bottom part of your body ie the Spleen...

One surgery in Canada can cost about $10K (10 thousand canadian dollars)

A visit to a doctor may cost less, but if it leads to unnecessary surgery you are now actually bankrupting yourself...Why? because contrary to popular belief, the gov't of Canada & OHIP KNOWS who spends the most on surgeries & who pays the most in taxes...If you contribute the least in taxes but spend the most on surgery then you may not be liked by the OHIP people...

For example...If you paid 4K in taxes last year but had a one month hospital stay last year then you should know a hospital stay used to cost $800 dollars a day for psychiatric at the Clarke Institute (now called CAMH Canadian centre for addiction & mental health or something like that)...

$800 X 31 days = $24,800.00 for one month stay in mental health facility...

Now if the staff are abusive to you or the food is terrible then they are cutting costs to you by half maybe so your stay will then only cost the country & your tax bill only $12,400.00
Now if they kill you because you paid only 4K in taxes but you opted for say a lumpectomy surgery or a ballon catheter kyphoplasty where they inject resin into the

cracks of your spine or your knees or whatever you have degraded due to excessive sports watching. playing or encouraging...

Then they are killing you because you paid in to OHIP $4K but your surgery that year cost $400K, or 200K if it sucked but was ok, or $100K if they got the job done but no nurses were nice to you...

So you got killed because you owe the surgeon & the hospital & Ohip & the gov't & your caregivers about maybe say $96K...

So if you or a friend died during unnecessary surgery in Canada you might think twice about suing...

Because you have shorted some very important kind people out of their livelihood...

Just because you paid your taxes doesn't give you the right to abuse the system...

Surgeons need to be paid just as much as gov't employees...

If you got a good Kyphoplasty surgery at Toronto general Hospital great...But I promise you it will be cheaper to go back to your Naturopath or Acupuncturist or TCM(Traditional Chinese medicine)doctor & nurses & herbs supplement stores than going in for another major surgery...Because the second time around you may not get that Mulligan...

A Mulligan means you got lucky once...It is a golf term...It means someone gives you a freebie once...

Mulligans don't happen more than once...

Miracles do...Mulligans no...

Don't push the system...

On a personal note: If a bug enters your personal parts (like your crotch or penis area), Ginseng tea will get it out...Ginseng...It is from the Ginger ROOT...It also comes in a gel Ginseng tea taste format...I had 8 Ginseng gel teas & 2 giant regular Ginseng teas at the Ginseng tea shop in the Village by the Grange across from OCADU-The Ontario College of Art & Design University...Then the bug that went up my crotch area left, later...It was a horrifying experience & I am so grateful for the Herb Depot & the TCM doctors there (father & daughter) for being patient with my hysteria...The new drugstore (Rexall??) at the corner of College & Spadina was also most patient & their cushy bench seats upstairs near where the pharmacists work were orange & placid inducing...Nice...

Pay out of pocket...Pay out of pocket...Pay out of pocket...

Welfare & unemployment insurance & relying on OHIP are for when you are in money trouble...

If you can, pay out of pocket for the better services of the private medical clinics like the Cleveland Clinic of the other one called um, MedCan I think...

Both lovely & good reviews from 3 separate people...

3 separate people who I spoke to directly & asked extensive questions-one was a political canvasser for the Progressive Conservatives...

On that note...

I support Olivia Chow for Mayor this October 2014 because she is female...

I support Guide Dogs for Israel because I love dogs & they help the visually & physically impaired so well...

I support weddings between a lady & a gentleman because that is what I know & like...

I support birthdays because it is good to be alive...

This does not mean that I don't support other causes or ideas or people or theories...

It just means that I have BIAS towards myself as we all do...

My BIAS is my bias & I like that...

'Don't take up a cross for another' means to look out for number one...

'By their fruits ye shall know them' means if the tamarind orange peel tastes good so is probably too the bartender who served it to you at Frank restaurant...

with the calamari...

dipped in milk...

rolled in chick pea flour...

rolled in tamarind orange peel gratings...

with sauteed onions...

with a glass of water freshly washed soaped glass...
after the Alex Colville exhibition at the AGO Art Gallery of Ontario...which was the best show Sari had ever seen up until now yesterday!

Memberships at the AGO get you reciprocal memberships at a bunch of other galleries outside the province of Ontario which is neat...

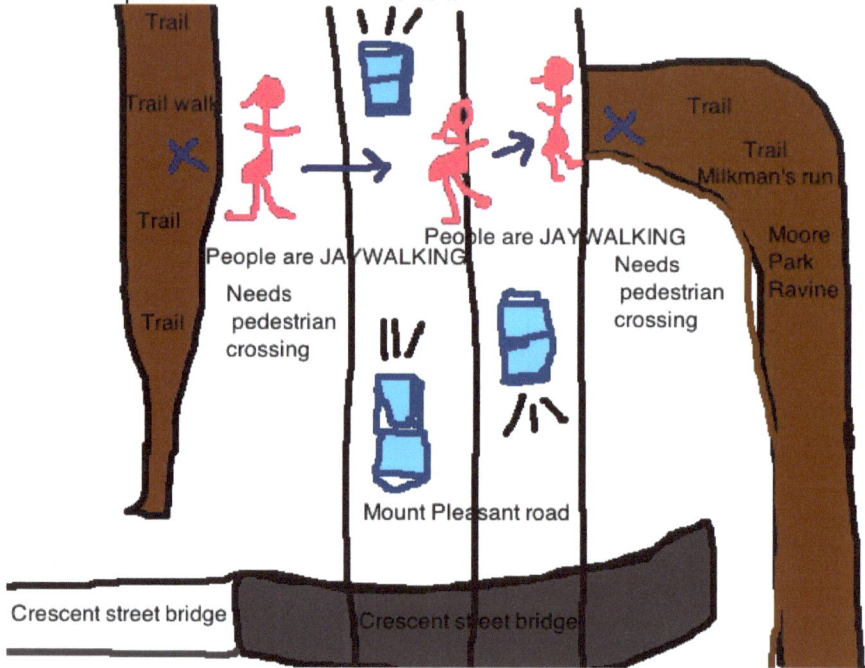

311

311

311

is the number # you call to speak to a CITY official in Toronto, Ontario, Canada...

They have been nice to me at least 4 times...out of 4...

That is 100% nice...Good ratio...

Drinking & driving is still illegal & I think all liquids can be dangerous there including coffee tea Kombucha or water...Falling asleep at the wheel can occur due to drinking too much liquid...Liver...Hydrogen...Plus element...Stop & pee to clear your liver & wake you up...

New tipping is a Pay it forward method because you have to pay often before you even drink your drink...This causes consternation amongst clients...It is better for bartenders though...

Watermark Cafe...Sommersby Cider, Apple juice, Cucumber salad with onions & DILL!

Shakey's Bar...Smirnoff vodka one shot, soda water, lime...

I thought they were just fine for cyclists...

High Park Zoo was not available for viewing to me because of construction at High Park near Grenadier restaurant...Best restaurant in a park for breakfast so far by far summers so far only...

Missing fingers:If a...?

a finger is made of-

bone-thyroid zinc + lead

blood thymus iron + manganese

cartilage(the joint part the bendy part)

skin Bismuth Colon Fluorine

then you need ALL of the ABOVE elements to regrow a NEW finger...

If the finger is the 4th finger missing then it involves the MAIN artery to the heart...

Tubes are made in the Kidneys...So add;

Kidneys Carbon + Nitrogen

If the heart is involved because you are SAD that you got your finger(s) cut off while sawing wood i construction or something then...

Add Heart Aurum(gold) & Potassium (bananas)...

Having a PET rabbit Caregiver is an exellent source of Aurum(gold because Rabbits have good hearts)...
Banana Bread is NOT the same things as just bananas...

A BLUE potato is not just a potato...A potato is Lead for the bones...A blue potato is actually Purple on the inside & has been bred with a BEET...A blue potato is thus Lead for the Bones Plus Nitrogen for the Neural or renal or whatever tubes in the body...

If you have lost an arm then you may have lost muscle...Muscles are made in the Lymph Node & Lung section...Lungs are like balloons & needles should not be stuck into them...A needle biopsy is into the lungs actually...It WILL deflate your lung balloon...A breast is just the top surface of the lung...Most needle biopsies by nature go into & through lung tissue by protocol...This causes holes in the lungs...promise...

Muscle then is Lung & Lymph Node Titanium & Aluminum...Eggs are an Aluminum...Cloves are a Titanium...

A better way to medicate the breast is via the armpits which are holey & you can put medicine there that will feed the lungs, lymphs & breast tissue & muscle...

Most deodorants including herbal ones are Aluminum based even if they just say marigolds or echinacea or cinnamon which are all Aluminum family...But the herbal ones are less so maybe safer if you have a lung infection...

Dogs are awesome friends...In Washington D.C. if you want a friend get a dog...Pretty much the same if you are disabled, or just not feeling well...Rent a Dog or Rent some Ducks or become a Dogwalker, BirdFeeder, or Catnapper in order to socialize more...

People will be amazed at your chameleon in the aquarium or the snake your brought to college...

**dyslexia among seniors due to lack of poohing due to fear of making a smell in the house due to fear of annoying caregivers due to caregivers muscling in on seniors' home & money & property & privacy etcetera...mercury excess in gallbladder...treat with epsom salt baths if you have time or (even?) better if in a rush half a tablespoon lemon juice with half a tablespoon olive oil drink fast...

Hire a cleaning lady to clean...Caregivers are not cleaning ladies...Nurses are not the same as caregivers...Babysitters are not free...Family members are not medical personnel but can be either better or worse or neutral when it comes to helping out...Just because someone is family doesn't mean they are safe with their sibling or other family member if that person is disabled...

Those who mind dont matter & those who matter dont mind A successful woman is one who can build a firm foundation with the bricks others have thrown at her. (This is a link to a Facebook Page I like...)

what follows is our App,

like, what I mean is, I have copied & pasted the Contents of our App into this book so people who cannot seem to access the app can sort of get an idea of what is in it...not everything copied & pasted, like for example, the Quizzes you don't get to see the answers but on the App you do... (Ha! encourages you to go see it online doesn't it?)

http://bwell.mobi/grove is a Desktop or Mobile device(ie: iPhone) application which means that it is like a book but smaller & organized so the content page is clickable...(like if when you read a real paper book you go to the contents page tap your finger on what you want to read about & the paper magically flips to that page–that is what an App is)...

Description(from the http://InfiniteMonkeys.com App market store)

Read Grove Body Part Chart:A Medical Arts Innovation, & Do it Yourself Medicine:A Repair Manual FREE! Two Canadian artists have re-defined the Medical Arts by creating a chart that tells you what your imbalance is, what its antidote is, & where to find that element in the real world...The body is broken down into 11 organs & each organ is shown to have 2 elements that must live in balance for health...Finally understand your own health! Simple yet powerful information! The first book explains the basics, & goes through many common ailments, their specific imbalance, & things in the real world that contain the element you need to rebalance your body...The second book gets into some more complicated problems, using the Grove Body Part Chart as well... Once you get the idea, you will be using these ideas to analyze things you have been told by doctors & remedies you have been given...For example, Cancer is a Calcium excess in the Adrenal Gland & its opposite element is Iodine...

Welcome

WELCOME

Home

Welcome...(Turn this

message

sideways on your Mobile

device

so it doesn't all get cut

off at

the sides!)

This is

GroveBodyPartChart

the MOBILE APP...

Since this is a DIY Medicine

Application, it is possible that

you are having a health problem

or you know someone who is...

I am very sorry to hear that...

I am here to help...

Here you will find a 23 minute

VideoTalk that explains my

very very basic medical chart...

Once you "get" that, you are

on your way...

Book 1 is called Grove Body

Part Chart:A Medical Arts

Innovation...

It explains the whole chart

better, & then tells you what

excess or imbalance is what

in which disease & where to

find its opposite element,

its antidote or remedy in the

real world...

In the 2nd Book, called Do

it Yourself Medicine:A repair

Manual, I talk about some

more complicated

imbalances

which cause diseases...

The books are full of great

art done by me! because

art is a great way to relax

your brain from all that

logical

thinking(read boring

thinking)

...

There is a movie called

RightBrain which is 10

minutes

in 3d animation also done

by

me, which really gets your

brain out of that too much

thinking mode...

Which might happen from

reading...

The Quizzes are fun to see

if you really got the books

into your head...

Plus it's a fast way to get

answers(because I cheated,

&

just give them to you, right

after I ask the questions)

:)

...

You can Contact me by

pressing the EMAIL

button icon,(it is a

Contact form made by

Wufoo, not a thingy that

opens up your email

server or anything

scary like that)-

& I totally will answer you

as fast as I can...(Be

prepared,

I am Canadian, so fast is

like the speed of snow

melting

here...)

There is an Amazon

page

for BOOK 1,

if you want to

have

a real book in your hands...

BOOK 2 has its own

page too...I can't link

those pages from inside

this APP, because

the pages will be too big

for people on mobile

devices & then they

will get either mad

or depressed when their screen

freezes up & crashes...

(Kindle versions as well as

Paperbacks are there for

both books)

Don't feel pressured to buy...

I love trees...

My married last name is

Grove

& I still love Mr. Grove very

much(& have been Mrs.

Grove

for over 17 years now!)...

You may be scared...

That's normal...

Fear is good...

It protects you from doing

stupid things...

You may be around alot of

doctors & nurses &

technicians

& they are all strangers &

they all apparently want to

see you naked & stick

needles

into you...

This is why fear is good...

You may just want to flee...

That may be a good idea...

Please don't let me be the

one to tell you to ignore

your

fears...

They are real...

The best I can do is give you

answers about medicine &

health that nobody else has

told you before because I

hadn't thought them up yet...

With these answers you will

have superpowers...

The superpower of being

smarter than everyone else

around you...

Now that you are going to

be smarter, you will be able

to make decisions about your

own health, FOR YOURSELF...

It's your body, why should

somebody else be the expert

on it?

If you think something about

something, & someone tells

you you are wrong about that,

because they went to this

school or that school, then

that makes you feel weak...

Weak is not good for your

immune system or health...

I want you to know that even

without reading my books or

watching my videos or

anything

at all, that you are the

EXPERT

of your own body...

I don't care how crazy

people

say your ideas are...

It's your body & your

ideas &

everybody else is just

wrong...

Ask alot of questions,

get a

second opinion, get a 3rd

opinion, in fact keep

getting

opinions until you get

one you

like...

Your health is the number

one

thing in your life...

This is not a time to get

the on

sale quickie price...

Beware of words like

"prophylactic surgery"...

Removing parts of your

body

is pretty final, especially

if

there isn't anything wrong

yet...

Genetics is a funny thing...

Your Mum could have a love

of peanut butter but you

can be born just

altogether hating peanuts...

So just cause a parent had

one thing doesn't mean you

will get it too...

Even if studies say so...

Because a genetic marker

can

be there & just do NOTHING

at all...

Sure you might have a

predisposition...

But if you figure out what

that

predisposition is exactly,

you

can STEER your boat away

from

that ICEBERG! I am here

to help...

Help you steer your boat

away

from an Iceberg...

Personally I think people

are

taking way too many drugs &

not feeding swans enough...

Personally I think that alot of

new diseases are caused

by all this drug

taking...

I like to feed swans in winter,

between November & April,

because it makes me happy

inside & it helps to save

their lives...

I think if more people did

stuff

for nature, for animals & trees

& fresh oxygen air, that more

people would be healthy &

happy...

My goal is to get people to

take

the power back from the so

called

experts including myself

(which

is a bit of a bind isn't it

philosophically) & Do it

Yourself their Medicine alot

more...

Ok I'm not saying to go

rogue...

I'm just saying that there

are some things we can do

& understand about health

that might be able to be done

without so much outside help...

Sari Grove, Tuesday February

4th, 2014 p.s.if you are a woman

then maybe a woman doctor

might be more comfortable

for you...If you are 85 years old,

you might prefer an 85 year

old doctor...If you speak

Spanish you might want a

doctor who is fluent in Spanish...

This is important...Don't be

afraid to say:"This is what

I am comfortable with &

this is not"...Don't be

afraid to run away...There

are some scary things about

medicine...If you want to

run away & live in Tijuana,

or Paris or Peru, then that

might be a really really fun

& good & healthy idea...Escape

is always a fun way out...bring

my books or this App...Just

in case you

missed something! :)

Technical Message:When you

go to read either of the Books,

it takes you to the

Smashwords page for

the book,

where

they are available as Pdfs,

Kindle mobi files, epub files,

read online, & a few other

types of file...(all free)

Kindle has a free

Mobile app for

if you are on

a Mobile device &

 want to read books easily...

get it...It's free...

You don't need to subscribe to

anything...But the Mobile

app makes the Books really

really more readable on a

Mobile device...

Like the difference between:

"No, I am

not going to bother" & "hey

this is fascinating stuff"...

(plus each book as a

paperback sells for like

over 40 dollars on Amazon,

so you are getting to read

them for free, so the trouble

is kinda worth it, dontcha

think?)(Note:The Smashwords

free Kindle versions are less

than 10 megabytes, whilst

the pay for Kindle versions

on Amazon are the full book

size-so the pictures might

be slightly better in the pay

for versions-but I use the free

versions myself to doublecheck

edits-so don't fret about it)...

Ok, that said, I will go on

to the next point...If you

do one of the Quizzes,

& then click

Submit, it takes you to

Grooveshark, which is a

free

music listening site...The

page is a singer songwriter

named Ryan Huston & you

can listen to some of his

songs there...(Ryan Huston's

song Do What You Love"

should be listened to,

if you can find it...)

I chose this

musician & this music

especially

for you...It is good &

meaningful

& right for all what we are

talking

about here on the

GroveBodyPartChart

App...

So give it a hear...

Now, Grooveshark will also

ask if you want their free

Mobile App too...get it...

The Mobile app means you

have music for free all the

time just by clicking that

button on your home screen...

Music is a good thing...get

the app...Commit to some

music listening...

The song "Thank You" is also

a good listen...

(Oh, here, I found his iTunes

page link...here it is...)

The other Quiz, when

you click

the word "Submit",

takes you to the video,

that

I made, as an entry,

to the Clinical trial

Patiet Engagement App

Challenge on

ChallengePost...

If this App wins a prize,

it would be neat to be

able to see

the actual video that was

used for the

contest...

Sari

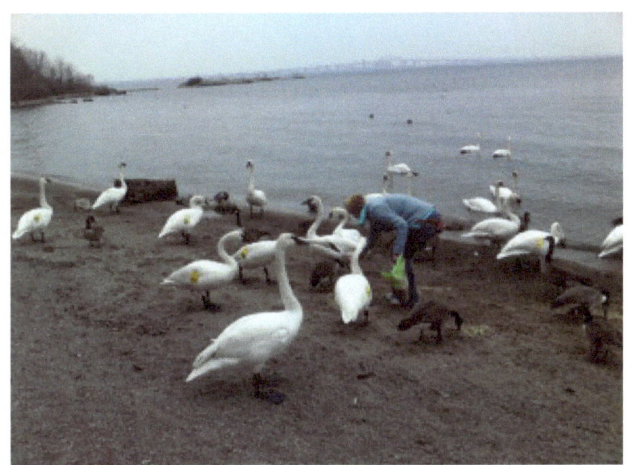

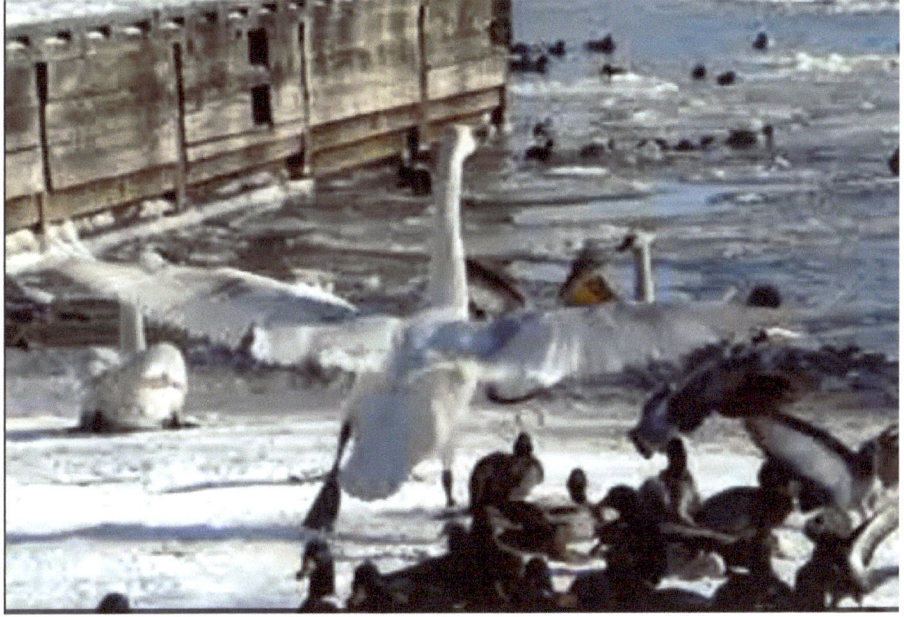

If you are on a device

that is

having trouble

reading the books,

go to the DOCS page,

& I have put there,

TEXT files of Book 1

& Book 2, which are tiny

files, UNformatted,

NO pictures, No charts,

But you should be able

to see & read these files...

When you get home or go

to a library, you can

then view

the longer versions

on a desktop

computer...

I have copies on

SMASHWORDS,

which are less than

10 megabytes,

& I have copies on Amazon,

which are in KINDLE

format,

as well as PAPERBACK

format...

The publishers I have

worked with

have discounted

the price of

publishing a bit, however,

be aware that not

every version

is free...That is because

both

 digital books & paper

books

have inherent material

costs

that are not related

to the

intellectual property

created by

the author...I do not earn

any money

from your purchases...

Any

royalties the publishers

might send

me might perhaps

recompense

me for the price of a donut

& coffee,

however, an author

cannot make

a living

from book sales if they

are forced

to give free versions,

due to OHIP expectations

created

by Canadian governments...

True story:Canadian

doctors

have been filling their

waiting rooms,

& seeing people who are

totally healthy

& well...

OHIP only pays when

you see someone...

So...They are seeing

someone...

Income levels are at

such an all time

low for doctors in Canada,

due to OHIP & the ban

of extra billing fees,

that doctors

have been forced to

get creative about

getting money back

from

an insurance company

that

seems to like holding on

to all that tax money...

Insurance used to

be called

Protection money in

Chicago,

& it was an operation

run by thugs

who'd break your

store window

if you didn't pay once

a week to a guy

named George...

Not sure why the Ontario

Health Insurance Plan

OHIP

would have been

expected to be

any different from George...

Before OHIP came in,

doctors could actually

earn a living...

Which is why today, the

pharmaceutical companies

have felt the

need to try to step up & fill

that gap...

At least someone is

stepping up...

The reason people often

like Clinical Trials is that

often the drugs &

treatment are free...

The reason Clinical Trials

are often free,

is that Physicians feel

sorry for

certain patients & set up

 a free type study,

really just to make it all

free...

For that person...

Which is why, if you

happen to be in one of

those benevolent

studies, that you should

stick with it...

Someone went to alot

of trouble to

try to heal you, & if you drop out

of the study, you are thwarting

some very good people who

maybe have a cure for what

ails you...

Sari Grove

Monday February 10, 2014

12:52 am

Sochi Olympics Russia

on tv right now,

who woulda thunk that?

1 Corinthians 13:1-3

New International Version

If I speak in the tongues

of men

or of angels, but do not

have love,

I am

only a resounding gong or

a clanging cymbal.

If I have the gift of prophecy

and can

fathom all mysteries and

all knowledge,

and if I have a faith that can

move mountains,

but do not have love, I am

nothing. If I

give all I possess to the poor

and give over

my body to hardship that

I may boast,

but do not have love, I gain

nothing.

p.s.The EMAIL button takes you

to a form where you can report

glitches or other problems with

this App...There is also a link

to the Smashwords page

for our in progress book 3,

which you can download,

& access in various less than

10 megabyte forms...Scroll

to the bottom of that page,

& there are Book 1,

& Book 2, also in

pdf, Mobi, Kindle, online read,

& other mobile

versions that are sure to suit

whatever you have...

EMAIL

Wufoo
Contact Form

TRANSLATE OUR BOOKS INTO ANY LANGUAGE BY VISITING THIS LINK–choose
language, then click HOME

When you click Submit, I get your Email address(which I do nothing with unless
you asked a question & wanted an answer...)
& your Message, & you get redirected to my Smashwords page where there are
Doc versions(less than 10 megabytes) of my two books, plus our 3rd book in
progress,

(also Kindle versions, Pdf, text & more)...Plus a Bio & Interview...Note:If you get
the Kindle app, the Kindle versions are really neat!

why this App was created–hint, a Challenge Post Competition!

Also, 50 recent blog posts that show the Research & Ideas behind our Grove
Health Science Book Series

Important thought:

Killing things is NOT the job of the Physician...There are other people who are better qualified to kill people(they are called surgeons)...The Hippocratic Oath includes mention of this...

My new line of Ground Coffee is called "Hammered" & it is...Hand hammered with a hammer, the irregular shape of the grounds makes for an asymmetrical coffee taste...If you pay extra, I will send you a video of my staff, hammering the coffee beans, while they whistle "I'd rather be a hammer than a nail", & are watched by a Hammerhead shark...

for at home desktop computer viewing in HTML5

If you are on an ANDROID device(65% of mobile users) or an iPhone(25% of mobile users) or a tablet or iPad(10% of mobile users), the Monkeys have APPS for you...

This APP, GroveBodyPartChart, is there too...

iTunes is waiting for me to stop updating builds of my App, so they can review it & put it in their iTunes APP store...

If they say no, then that's ok too, because you don't need to go to the iTunes App store, or the Google Play app store, or even the new Windows app store, because if you just type bwell.mobi/grove into the address bar of your browser, you get to the APP...

(in the interim)Mobile Opera offered us a place in their Application store, so we typed I agree into that!

So if you don't want middlemen or middlewomen or just middling, save GroveBodyPartChart to your Home screen (you get the awesome SWAN icon), & be done with the middles...(except the Oreo middles, I cannot live without them...Sorry for eating them all out then putting the unmiddled cookies back into the package...It wasn't my fault, they were DOUBLESTUFF! In my defense...)

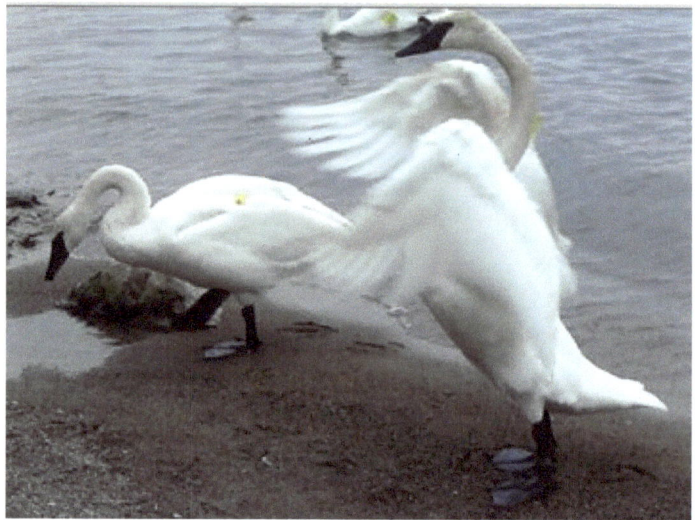

A Trumpeter swan displays! (if you click the arrows on the picture you can scroll through our Flickr account of pictures–our art!)

smaller versions of our 2 books(& the Galley Proof copy of our 3rd in progress book)!, less than 10 MB, in pdf, Kindle, mobi, text, & more... You need the Kindle app to download the Kindle versions...(but worth bothering doing)...

My gift to you is a sketch of some white Amaryllis flowers that you can download & have my permission to print-the file is big enough to make a 2 ft. x 3ft. print

Here is a sneak peak at our 3rd Book WHICH IS STILL BEING WRITTEN!!!

Algae+Rhythm, Algae-Rhyme:Apt surgical rotation app...Book 3 preview (warning unedited with raw parts)

1   **Message** *

    This field is required.
2   **Email Address**

    We won't share this with strangers.

VIDEO (it's 23:46 minutes long, sorry)...

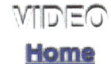

Home

Wufoo
Quiz 1
Grove Body Part Chart

This is a different kind of Quiz...

I GIVE you the answers...

So EVERYONE gets 100% right!

Now YOU know what the answers to these tough questions are!

You're welcome!

Be well!

When you click Submit, I get an email with all the answers that have been selected...(nothing else)

When you click SUBMIT, you get taken to a Vimeo page which is part of my CHANNEL GroveGrove & you get to watch the short film that was the entry video for the competition that this App was made for...The best is the music, the song FLY AWAY by Chantelle Barry, from her album SONGBIRD...That is a good song!

(but back to the fact that I get a copy of your Quiz answers when you click submit)

But why do I need that if all the answers are right already?

The "OTHER" box has a TEXT field...

if anyone has a different opinion than me about what is the right answer & feels the need to tell me that, PLEASE put your answer in the OTHER text field & choose the OTHER button too...

When you click Submit, I will get your ideas...

If I am indeed wrong & you are indeed right, not only can I correct the Quizzes but I can edit the books & we can help to make the world a better place...

So that is why there is an OTHER box...

(Please don't use the text field to write something mean or gross or sexy...I am a shy Virgo who blushes when the wind blows from the West...I have never eaten spam either & don't really want any thanks though...)

YOU ARE A SUCCESS!

Did you know that being in pain can really affect how you treat others?

Injuries can really affect how you treat people around you...If you have hurt yourself, make it a priority to get rest & relaxation & spend some time on the healing...Don't put it off...Popping painkillers & going back to work with an injury can hurt your business, your relationships, your family, your friends, & you can even cause yourself further injury...

Visit Audio Mp3 30Mb

above is secret link to mp3 file 30 MB how the grovebodypartchart works...

This link

Visit Doc file book 1

takes you to a Smashwords version of GroveBody Part Chart:A medical Arts Innovation

Book 1...

Then negotiate with whatever you get because I am watching the Sochi Olympics figure skaters now!

Go figure!

We are writing Book 3 right now, this is a working version>

QUIZ(correct answers have an asterisk beside them)...

1   **Parkinson's disease is an excess of what element in the Spleen?**

Zinc

Phosphorus*

Calcium

Other

2   **Cancer is an excess of what element in the Adrenal Gland?**

Magnesium

Calcium*

Aluminum

Other

3 Epilepsy is an excess of what element in the Colon?

Fluorine*

Titanium

Hydrogen

Other

4 Arthritis is an excess of what element in the Gallbladder?

Magnesium*

Manganese

Sulphur

Other

5 Downs' Syndrome is an excess of what element in the Kidneys?

Zinc

Aluminum

Carbon*

Other

6   Alzheimer's disease is an excess of what element in the Lungs &
    Lymph Nodes?

Carbon

Mercury

Titanium*

Other

7   Bipolar disorder is an excess of what element in the Thyroid?

Sulphur

Iron

Zinc*

Other

8   Hypertrophic Cardio Myopathy is an excess of what element in the
    Heart?

Potassium*

Aurum

Titanium

Other

9 High blood pressure is an excess of what element in the heart?

Iron

Aurum*

Aluminum

Other

**10 Asthma & Tuberculosis are an excess of what element in the Lung &
Lymph nodes?**

Phosphorus

Titanium

Aluminum*

Other

11 Multiple Sclerosis is an excess of what element in the Thyroid Gland?

Lead*

Iron

Aluminum

Other

12 Diabetes is an excess of what element in the Pancreas?

Phosphorus

Selenium

Sulphur*

Other

13 ADHD Autism is an excess of what element in the Gallbladder?

Selenium

Magnesium

Mercury*

Other

14 The Common Cold & Chronic Fatigue Syndrome are an excess of what element in the Liver?

Sulphur

Oxygen

Hydrogen*

Other

15 Kidney Blockages feature an excess of what element in the Kidneys?

Aurum

Nitrogen*

Carbon

Other

Quiz 2

Wufoo
Quiz 2

Do it Yourself Medicine

You will get 100% right on this Quiz...

I promise...

How do I know that?

Because I gave you all the right answers...

The key is to learn them, so you know them...

Might come in handy sometime...

Be well!

When you click Submit, I get an email with all the answers that have been selected...

(I don't get anything else, no cookies, or information about your computer or anything, not even your email address if you don't put it in)...

Songbird–the vocalist who did the song Fly Away for our competition entry video for this Challenge Post challenge

Submit takes you to the iTunes Mobile page for singer songwriter CHANTELLE BARRY who is awesome & has some songs for you to listen to right now just snippets that will groove your soul & rock you in your shoes & float your boat...

Ryan Huston is the male vocalist, whose song Do What you Love was the original entry song for our video...Indeed, one can still see that video on our Youtube or our Vimeo channels... GroveCanada on Vimeo

Visit Ryan Huston on Grooveshark

But why do I need that if all the answers are right already?

The "OTHER" box has a TEXT field...

if anyone has a different opinion than me about what is the right answer & feels the need to tell me that, PLEASE put your answer in the OTHER text field & choose the OTHER button too...

When you click Submit, I will get your ideas...

If I am indeed wrong & you are indeed right, not only can I correct the Quizzes but I can edit the books & we can help to make the world a better place...

So that is why there is an OTHER box...

(Please don't use the text field to write something mean or gross or sexy...I am a shy Virgo who blushes when the wind blows from the West...I have never eaten spam either & don't really want any thanks though...)

Success! Thanks for doing this Quiz! You get an A++

YOU ARE TOTALLY AWESOME! really!

Question:

Have you ever thought you heard voices? (Don't worry if you do, it is more common than you think & you are not nuts!)

Here is an explanation of that phenomenon:

Soundwaves are large...Thoughtwaves are smaller...Our brains are designed to hear soundwaves...When you get a concussion, your brain swells up...Sometimes you end up with a permanent swelling, edema, that stays that way...The swelling makes your brain smaller...If it makes your brain smaller anywhere near the hearing area, it affects what kind of waves you can hear...Because a concussed brain is now smaller, sometimes only the smaller thoughtwaves get through, where they did not before...So when you are very close to a person or an animal(people are animals but anyways), the smaller concussed brain can hear the tiny thoughtwaves in the other creature...if the brain heals & goes back to normal size, the larger waves come through again, &

the brain is no longer able to process the tiny thought waves...Many people who were once concussed can hear the smaller thoughtwaves, but don't admit it because they think it's crazy...It's actually scientific...

Visit Algae+Rhythm, Algae-Rhyme:Apt surgical rotation app

The link takes you to the WORKING version of our THIRD BOOK...(secret)

Algae+Rhythm, Algae-Rhyme:Apt surgical rotation app in Paperback

Quiz(answers have asterisk beside them)

1   **Which answer contains the greatest amount of manganese?**

Pumpkin Seeds*

Pyrite Beads

Oranges

Other

2   **Which body part processes iron?**

Thyroid

Lungs & Lymph Nodes

Thymus*

Other

3   Which element lowers blood sugar in the Pancreas?

Water

Garlic*

Fresh Air

Other

4   Which element can cause memory loss, schizophrenia & Alzheimer's?

Calcium

Magnesium

Titanium*

Other

5   Asthma is an excess of what element in the Lungs & Lymph Nodes?

Mercury

Lead

Aluminum*

Other

6 Which element corrects Parkinson's disease?

Titanium

Zinc

Copper*

Other

7 Which element corrects Cancer?

Iodine*

Fluorine

Calcium

Other

8   Epilepsy is caused by an excess of which element in the Colon?

Bismuth

Fluorine*

Mercury

Other

9   Joint Pain & Arthritis are an excess of what element?

Magnesium*

Mercury

Zinc

Other

10 The Common Cold & Chronic Fatigue Syndrome are an excess of which element?

Oxygen

Iodine

Hydrogen*

Other

11 Which food contains the highest amount of Iodine?

Green Beans

Seaweed*

Carrots

Other

12 Which answer contains the most Zinc?

Alcohol

Marijuana

Cigarettes*

Other

13 Which element lowers iron levels in the Thymus?

Magnesium

Manganese*

Titanium

Other

14 Which thing contains the most amount of mercury that builds cartilage in the gallbladder?

Cheese

Potato Chips

Bacon*

Other

15 Which element contains alot of Oxygen to treat the common cold?

Beets

Peanuts

Goji Berries*

Other

http://www.smashwords.com/books/view/349426 Grove Body Part Chart on Smashwords (smaller tiny versions free for your Kindle iPhone app)...
About Sari Grove
Grove Canada, or GroveCanada, is a registered business in Canada, owned by two partners, Joseph & Sari Grove & their cats B'Elanna & Jadzia Grove...(Which would make it 4 partners actually, but on paper it only mentions the two humans...But who said paper was the last word?) Much help has also arrived from reading other people's books, especially thanks to the book called The Philosopher & the Wolf by Mark Rowlands...That is how I solidified my ideas about Parkinson's & the Spleen...Please go online to read more about GroveCanada...Thanks for reading, Sari

https://vimeo.com/81439856 (our 3D animated film on http://www.Vimeo.com)

The award winning film based on the bestselling book...

from **Sari Grove** PLUS 8 months ago **ALL AUDIENCES**
3d animation apprentice:Bolakale Lukman
2013 reel Joseph & Sari Grove Medical Arts...
made with Blender 3d animation software...
audio made in Garageband for mac ...
Editing done in SIMPLEMOVIE...
DVD burn on Lacie DVD burner with new firewire converter cable from Apple...(Mac changed their firewire cable pin holes on their Snow Leopards, so getting this 6 pin to 9 pin converter cable

saved my .....!Thank Goodness Apple store's customer service was willing to go the extra mile to figure all that out for me!)
The two books are on my website at grovecanada.ca & you can read them both there as PDF files...
This film is the result of a year's work, 2013, learning Blender 3d animation software in order to make a movie about my Medical theory...
It became two books, with stills from my animation work...
But if you are interested in seeing the work behind the stills from the book, watch this!
The award winning film based on the bestselling book:DO IT YOURSELF MEDICINE:A REPAIR MANUAL

http://www.smashwords.com/books/view/388051 Do It Yourself Medicine:A Repair Manual

1   Series: *Grove Health Sciences*, Book 2
By Sari Grove

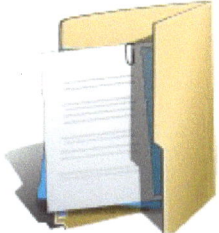

1

2 Grove Body Part Chart:A Medical Arts Innovation

This is Book 1...Just text...No charts or pictures or colour...But it's a small file & it will give you an idea...When you get home switch to your desktop...This version is for on the road reading...

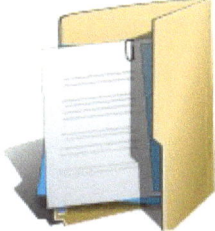

3

4 DIY Medicine TXT file no format 410 kilobytes

Tiny file of Book 2 for free no formatting of text but only 410 kb for those on really old mobile devices that can't download or see the bigger files...

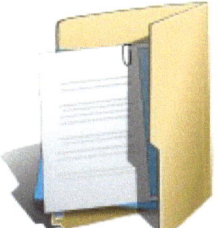

5

6 Algae+Rhythm, Algae-Rhyme:Apt surgical rotation app

Sat Feb 22nd 2014 3:51 pm et Bobsleigh team fell over, this book should help fix...emerg.(Working version only of Book 3)!

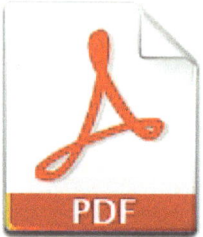

7

8 Transcript of the Audio speech from the Videotalk

If you don't have time to watch the whole Videotalk, or just don't feel like it, I typed out the audio into this file so you can read quickly how the GroveBodyPartChart works right here...The file after this one has a picture of the GroveBodyPartChart...

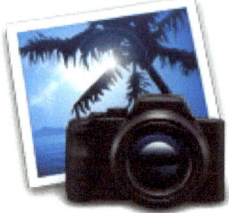

9

10 GroveBodyPartChart

This is what the back our business card looks like...It's the original GroveBodyPartChart...Refer to this chart when reading the audio transcript above...It encapsulates the whole medical theory the Grove Health Sciences series is based on...

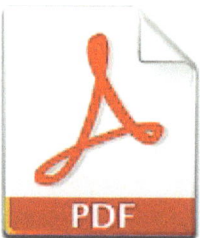

11

12 The original GroveBodyPartChart Image map

Drawn by artist Sari Grove, this was an early try at mapping out the GroveBodyPartChart in a comprehensible way...The info is still good & useful!

Menu

Messages
More Info
Send to a friend

Messages
Home

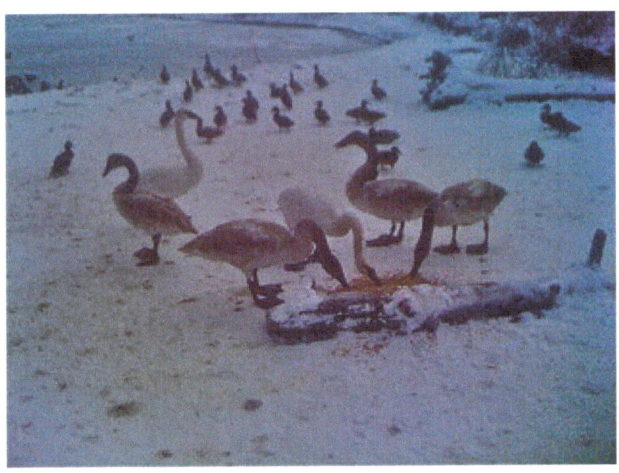

Hi...I'm Sari Grove...I built this App, Grove Body Part Chart, but I also wrote the books that are here...If you have any questions, feel free to write to me at grove@sent.com

So what you see when you open the App are a bunch of swan icons...Each one takes you to a different place...

There are 2 Book icons...Each one leads you to our Smashwords page for that book, where you can choose what kind of Free download you want of the book...

The books are:

(1)Grove Body Part Chart:A medical Arts Innovation

(2)Do It Yourself Medicine:A Repair Manual

There is now a 3rd book available to you for free called:

(3)Algae+Rhythm, Algae-Rhyme:Apt Surgical Rotation App

These are the 3 books of the Grove health Science series & should probably be read in order...

There is a VideoTalk that explains the basics of the Chart...Once you"get" the chart, the rest of your life's decisions about your health will seem so much simpler...

There is a 3d animated film that is about 10 minutes long...This should relax your brain if you seem to be seeing smoke coming out of your ears from too much left brain thinking...

The 2 Quizzes might seem daunting, so I GIVE you the answers...

This App was created for patients undergoing treatments in Clinical trials...So the welcome message will seem targeted to them...But, for anybody going through a health problem, this App will work...My guess is that people seek out health information when there is a problem...When things are ok, not so much...

The swans are because I like to feed Trumpeter swans between November & April, our winter months in Toronto...They are part of a restoration program & don't know how to migrate yet, so they need the food...But it has changed my winters...My winters are now such happy times I look forward to them...If you have long winters, I encourage you to go out & feed waterbirds...From your hand to their bills...Wild bird seed is great...It will save your life even more than it saves theirs...

Thanks for being here,

Sari Grove

p.s. paperback versions of our books are on Amazon if you want a keepsake...(but they are not free, sorry)... :(

More Info
Home

You can find me at
grovecanada.ca

or write me directly at
grove@sent.com

(Sari Grove)

BE WELL!

==
Created with the Infinite Monkeys self-publishing platform.
Want to make your own mobile app? Try it for free at:
www.monk.ee

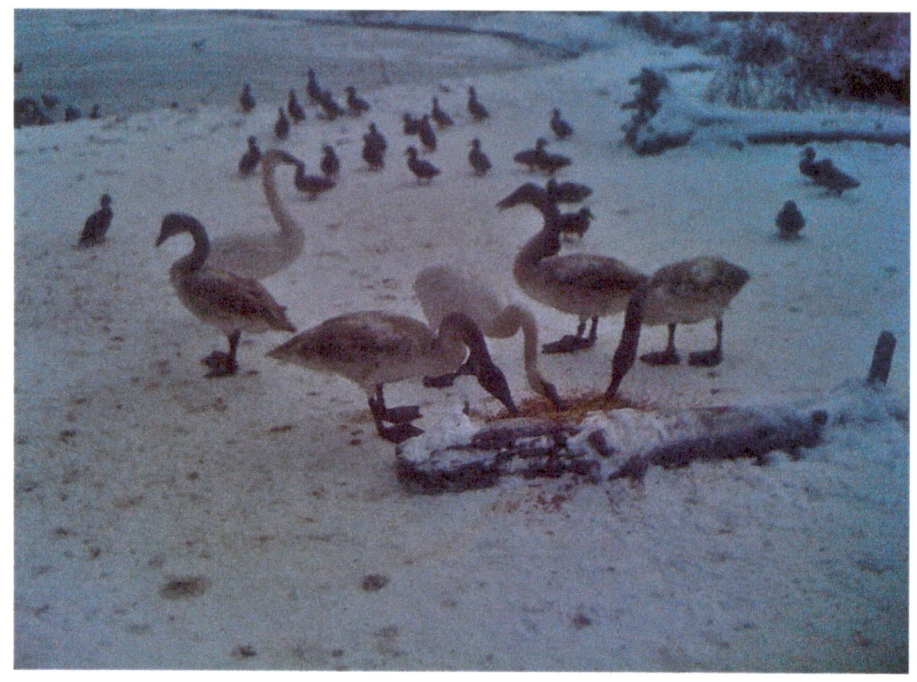

Send to a friend grove@sent.com

Check out this great app: http://bwell.mobi/grove

end of app

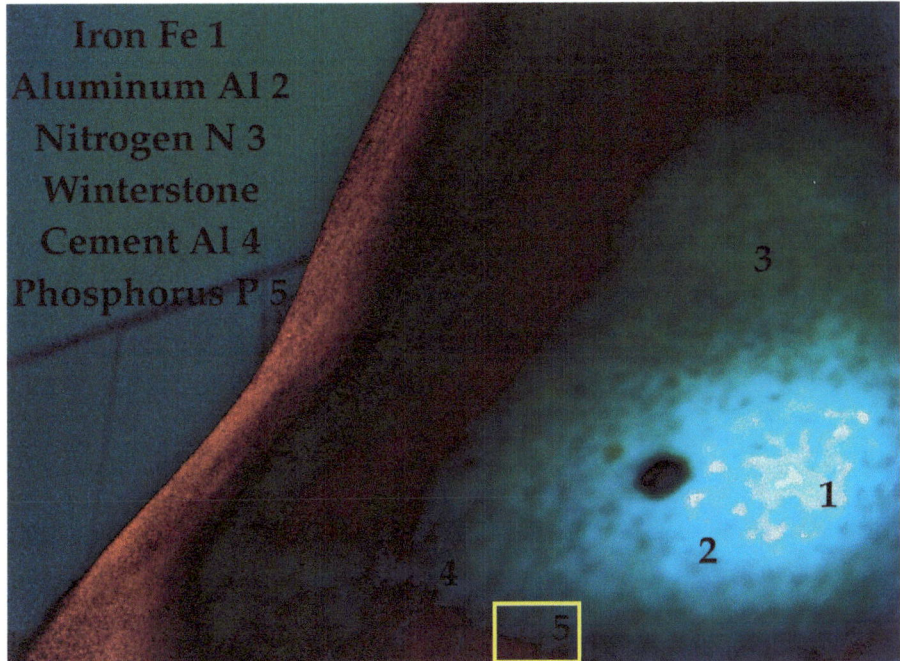

Iron Fe 1
Aluminum Al 2
Nitrogen N 3
Winterstone
Cement Al 4
Phosphorus P 5

Lump Aug. 31st, 2014 Progress Report;

Stress makes it worse due to constriction of Kidneys causing Nitrogen levels to rise...

1 is Iron Fe the SHINY white reflective stuff in the very centre of the lump...

2 is the Blue area around the shiny white & is the Aluminum Al which is maybe from eating eggs which are an Aluminum family thing...(Note Aluminum things patch holes up in the Lung Lymph Node area so this is not altogether bad if you have holes in your lungs from a breast Biopsy which is 2 holes actually)...

3 N Nitrogen is the green colour I think...Beets are a Nitrogen as are Genetically Modified Organisms & include all Glutens like pizza crust... (Some Organic Olive Oil Carbon C in a cup with some Apple Cider Vinegar

a Zinc Zn drunk quickly gets rid of Nitrogen blocks quickly by making you poop pooh)...

4 There is a dark formation like screws(hard to see sorry) which I know are the Cloves a Titanium Ti I swallowed...Cloves are a spice that are hard & small & shaped like a mushroom...If you swallow them & you have a hard piece of Concrete Aluminum Al in your lung, in your lump, the Titanium will be attracted to the Concrete Aluminum Al & will start to try to dissolve it...In your DIY Mammogram picture you will be able to see the Cloves turn SCREW shaped at their ends as they attack the Concrete...

Marijuana fume is in the air at Kensington market beside the music bar called Graffiti...(To the left is a bakery)...Marijuana fume is also a strong Titanium Ti which dissolves Aluminum concrete Al in the Lung...Strong Warning:If you inhale marijuana fume(which to be honest I think is really just in the Clove family), you WILL experience Memory loss...It is NOT sufficient by itself to remove your whole Lump so if you Just take marijuana fume my casually walking through Kensington market & just breathing normally, you WILL FORGET to do the other parts of your protocol...But it will help with dislodging the Cement dust or hard cement in your lung...(That maybe started this whole lump thing to begin with...Not)

I had some success with Kale, Spinach, PIneapple, Orange Juice(One whole Quart for $17.98) at the Loblaws at Bathurst & St. Clair North side East side...) I drank the whole quart almost in one shot in the middle of one of my "daily"(I cheat) 10 kilometere(6 mile) walks...The pressure of the flowing Hydrogen water liquid PUSHED the Winterstone cement concrete Aluminum OFF my inner Lung tissue...How do I know? I could feel it...(But be aware that Liquids like Hydrogen Water in Juices will make the lump swell up, so just eat a pinch of Raw saffron an Oxygen to REDEHYDRATE after trying the water pressure push method...

Note: DIY Biofeedback just means tuning yourself in to what you are doing & how it is affecting your body...Truly focussing on a body part or action helps you to know what is happening inside your body...No machines needed...Take notes after...It will help you to remember...

The purple edge is Phosphorus P which is hardly there because I boiled some Licorice root powder a Copper Cu with some Wheatgrass powder a

Copper Cu with a Splenda packet a Potassium K & some water a Hydrogen H...

Phosphorus is like mold which makes a "Cancer" grow or spread or whatever & is what makes it dangerous or malignant...I use Licorice root to revert the mold back to normal...That is called Phenotypic reversion-malignant to benign...

Jennifer Lopez is correct in saying that lukewarm water goes down easier than cold...Especially after your daily 10 kilometer walk...(Walks include breaks & going to the Alex Colville exhibition at the AGO Art Gallery of Ontario a blockbuster show by the best darn artist Canada has evah (yes EVAH) produced...

After the needle biopsy I had some water going into my lungs instead of esophagus...This is due to lack of pressure in the Lungs because a needle biopsy makes 2 HOLES in your LUNGS...

Toenail fungus responds very well to Vitamin D3 drops but take too many & you go Bipolar...Take too few & you will get bored & think it doesn't work...Fungus is Lead Plomb Pb on the Periodic Table...

Formaldehyde & Silicon Si & Mercury Hg & Salt NaCl are all in the Mercury family on the Grove Body Part Chart...(The picture below or on the next page if you are on a Kindle app on your iPhone is an earlier version of the business card chart which had drawings made in Blender 3d animation shareware freeware...That early series is part of show at WAMSOC (yes sounds like Wham! Sock!) which stands for the Women's Art Museum Society of Canada, & yes if you look for Sari Grove the show is all there online now & for history too which means a long time...http://www.wamsoc.ca)

Women's Art Museum Society of Canada - Edmonton, AB - Non ...

Women's Art Museum Society of Canada, Edmonton, AB. 86 likes.
Dedicated to preserving women's visual heritage.
https://www.facebook.com/pages/Womens.../134673196598463

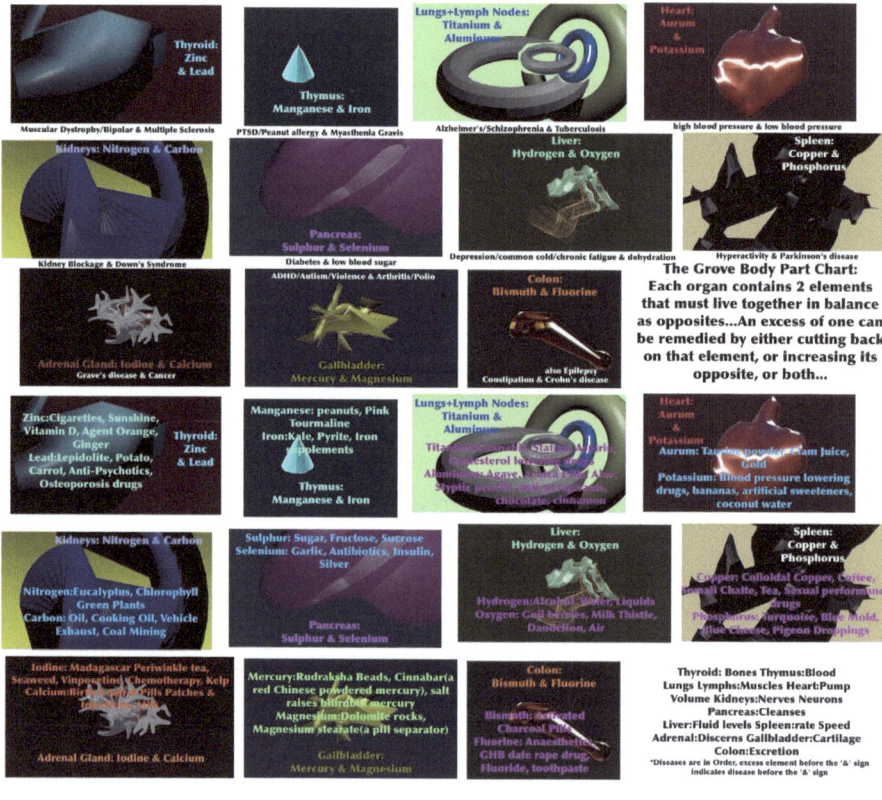

10% of an item can be copied for Library use in Canada...

Asking someone's religion as a work related question as put to a
Canadian is illegal which is why entering Israel if you are a Canadian is
dangerous...(They ask what religion you are before letting you on an

airplane...This question is illegal to Canadians who are there on work-related adventures)...

Two wrongs do not make a right...

It is illegal to change your name in Canada...Unless you get a permit...

Leaded fuel from airplanes or cars can cover wide spreads of territory in once nice places in Toronto...This looks like & is a Black fungus...Take Vitamin D3 50,000 International Units IU once a week or as needed...Be aware this can cause Bipolar symptoms...50,000 IU is 50 times the amount you will normally get in a drugstore...(You can also stick these tiny capsules between your toilet tank & your toilet in the tiny crack where they join to kill black fungus there...) Vitamin D3 is a Zinc Zn that comes in many forms but the vegetable glycerin base liquid drops work best for inner toenail fungus but cost way more than the capsules...But the capsules work too just slower it seems...The oily Carbon vegetable glycerin base seems to help the D3 travel & absorb better...Maybe drink your capsules emptied open & dissolved in organic olive oil to make them absorb better?

Drugstore brands will give you 1,000 Iu...You need to take 50 of those to get a result that you will see fast enough not to get bored of taking them if you are a Torontonian who gets bored easily or has ADD from people in boats dumping their poop toilet water directly into Lake Ontario instead of Legally taking the toilet tank to a Marina tank & the Marina tank gets given to the Water filtration people for cleaning the proper right way...

Licorice root absorbs way better in that alcohol base but that is expensive like almost 20 dollars a day if you want the Phosphorus mold P to stop spreading fast...Also sometimes you get just alcohol & not much licorice root so you have to buy from a reputable supplier & not go cheap about this...Botanica & St. Francis are very very good...You get what you pay for here...

Pho is a broth soup which you put fresh lemongrass & fresh Mint leafs into & bean sprouts...You can get Vegan broth at the Vietnamese restaurant at Ossington & Dundas south of Dundas towards Queen but on the East side of the road & tiny & good price & I know the owner & he has been cooking for 30 years & in Montreal La Vientiane is where I used to go for Lemongrass soup & that was amazing too!

Note:Tofu is a Bean which has been pulverized into a mash that gets shaped into little brick shapes...I love Tofu but it is a Phosphorus thing because the Nitrogen bean degrades down in the processing of it...Down the chart it goes as it degrades from Nitrogen to Sulphur(Sugar) to Hydrogen(Water) to Calcium(Milk) to Phosphorus(cheese)...So Tofu has maybe all of those Plus elements inside...

But Tofu may be the lesser of all the evils if you are at a Vietnamese restaurant & are ordering Pho soup with the fresh lemongrass leafs & the fresh mint leafs...Because Chicken or Beef Pho might have Iron in it which is hard to get rid of, & don't forget MANGANESE is what you use to do that...

Music at Graffiti bar in Kensington market-like Spadina west of Bathurst towards Ossington...Near where the Herb Depot store is with the TCM doctors who are really Chinese & really are Doctors...Ok, so music...
The band was playing IN TUNE & were hot & I could feel the metal strings pulsing through my chest as the electric guitars & basses & singing & microphone amplification pulsed...This caused intense lung stimulation & felt really really good & cleansing...Plus it made me happy & I bopped slightly sang a bit & clapped a little & that was good & free fro the cornerside of the road...

Also in Kensington is "One Heart" store which I went into to show the owner from Guatemala my Argentinian Rhodochrosite Manganese Heart stone on a silver Selenium chain...But if a Dolphin freezes to death on the beach of Newfoundland then his heart might be made of Rhodochrosite Manganese due to lack of Iron food because people are fishing all his small fish food off the coast of Newfoundland illegally...So know that mineral jewellery comes from somewhere & maybe limit your jewellery to things that are medicinal & maybe not from dolphins...The owner of One Heart said that if all that was true maybe the Dolphin died naturally if it froze to death because in Canada that is how things die here...That would mean if my rock is from that source I am off the hook polotically correct speaking but I still feel funny & have a pit in my stomach a little if that is where rhodochrosite might come from...My heart pendant came from ebay.ca from California but maybe a dolphin died there & became a rock that a jeweller decided to make into a stone pendant...But maybe the Dolphins from France loved me so much they left me that as a thank & an sort of inheritance? In Bordeaux in Cap Ferret the dolphins played with me...& my French dentist friend too of course who seemed to know them well as family there...& who also drove the boat because it was his boat & he knew the way through the sailboats that really sail with no motor needed & the island which was really uninhabited really with nobody there & nothing development at all at all...Je me souviens...That is the motto on the Quebec licence plates...Cars...That is another topic for discussion & guilt...

On the subject of guilt Robin Williams died & I saw Eddie Murphy at Kensington market & got to talk to him...I would have laughed just like him to show him my fandome but I have 2 stupid looking chips in my 2 front teeth bonding that make my teeth look like hooker teeth...So I couldn't do my Eddie Murphy laugh impression...Darn...

Gilson Lubin is a Canadian comic who is actually funny on a regular basis but his work is explicit so be aware of that...I think those tv roasts where they insult each other in explicit ways are totally disgusting but I guess comedians are really broke because jokes are so easily passed along for free on the internet...

Rod Stewart maybe was playing music on Bay street near to the new Four Seasons Hotel on the street & I think that is also because the internet has maybe killed income for musicians...

In the near future artists will be the new computer geek nerd genius in terms of money & we will all be filthy rich...Blessed are the poor (in spirit too) for they shall inherit the earth...New Testament I think...

Walked 10 km yesterday so am doing this writing today...Sari Grove on a Sunday...

Lung & Lymph Nodes=Titanium(Minus element)+Aluminum(...   Sari Grove   Today, 11:47 AM

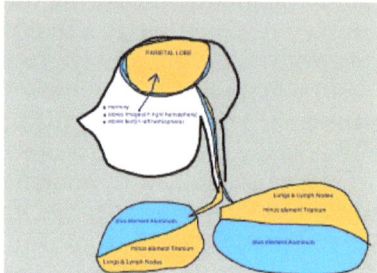

http://www.grovecanada.com/blog/2013/10/parietal-lobe-lungs-lymph-nodes-memory.html

THE PARIETAL LOBE:If the left frontal lobe is the Lead(plomb) element, & the right Frontal lobe is the Zinc element, THEN one might posit the RIGHT PARIETAL lobe (Lung & lymph node system) is the TITANIUM element, & the LEFT PARIETAL lobe is the Aluminum system...Seeing as the PLUS elements line up on the Grove Body Part Chart, & the Minus ones too...(Aluminum & Lead are both PLuses...)Note:The first element on the cover chart above is the Plus, all the way down...The second one is the Minus...(If I am right , that explains that the Titanium right Parietal lobe controls the left side of the body, the "artistic side" the IMAGES side, & the Aluminum element LEFT side of the Parietal lobe controls the numbers side, the accountant in all of us...

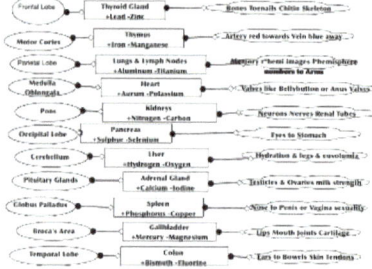

Lungs Lymph Nodes

= Too much Titanium (a Minus Element): Alzheimer's, Schizophrenia, Fear Panic Anxiety(Attacks), Memory Loss short medium or long term, Cerebral Palsy congenital, Hyperhidrosis/Sweatyness, Amnesia
Note:Anxiety is actually related to memory loss, as are panic attacks-yo are trying to do a task or plan your day, say while driving to work, & you are having trouble remembering all the tasks you need to do, then the anxiety begins, later it can develop into a panic attack-it is a fear that you cannot perform-this is all a Titanium excess in the Lung Lymph Node system...

Lungs & Lymph Nodes:

 Too much Aluminum (a Plus Element): Tuberculosis, Cystic Fibrosis,
Asthma...Warnings:People with Asthma(an Aluminum excess) often overmedicate their asthma medications(which are Titanium

Weird things that happened to me...

***drugged ice cube found at Aroma restaurant west of Spadina on Bloor North side in toronto ontario canada...Drug was anaesthetic propofyl-like fluorine ghb date rape drug...J.H. familial was handler that put ice cube(foggy look to ice cube is the fluorine) Sunday Aug 31 , 2014...Meal cost $13.50 no tipping was allowed...Ice cube was buried in Peach(berry) Iced tea drink...Red lentil soup with hot peppers capsaicin old, salad raw onions, raw shredded carrots, salad greens raw, olive oil on side in plastic cup, lemon slices(not wedges as stated) with seeds fine...Dosage of fluorine drug was so intense, after a 5 km walk, I had to buy antidote Prohibition Bitters containing strong dose smoke ash wood burnt in alcohol base $26.50 with other ingredients(licorice, hibiscus, etc.) Bismuth is antidote to fluorine drug...Took 2 dropperfuls yesterday after being drugged...Pupils were fixed & unmoving & smaller than normal & paralyzed...After Bitters (bought from BYOB on Queen street west of Bathurst east of Ossington) pupils immediately began dilating again...Left side of body was more affected than right side...Heart being monitored & taurine will be administered to avoid hemmorhagic heart attack...J.H. suspected of terrorist action drugging me at Aroma restaurant...Cell group at AGO Art gallery of Ontario committed act of terrorism this last week during Alex Colville exhibit...Works were defiled by 5 security guards who farted on purpose near to nude paintings & archival works...5 men in cell group, one had some sort of cicatrice scar at back of neck like some sort of operation had been done at the spinal cord or medulla oblongata area where the heart control is located...Timing of both these events seem attached to Royal Canadian Airshow of unmanned planes flying overhead during CNE canadian national exhibition...Suspected cohorts of J.H. stockbroker family are S.M. internet professionelle & C.S. military police officer...

follow-up: Pufferfish missing a spike seen at aquarium in bar on Queen west of University Avenue...Stealing by 3 daughters of Far East background in "It " store type location on corner of Queen, same peripherals as Salvation Army location but cleaner...Father seen sitting outside on balcony of store waiting for "get" of products...Spy type operation stealing intellectual property of Canadian...

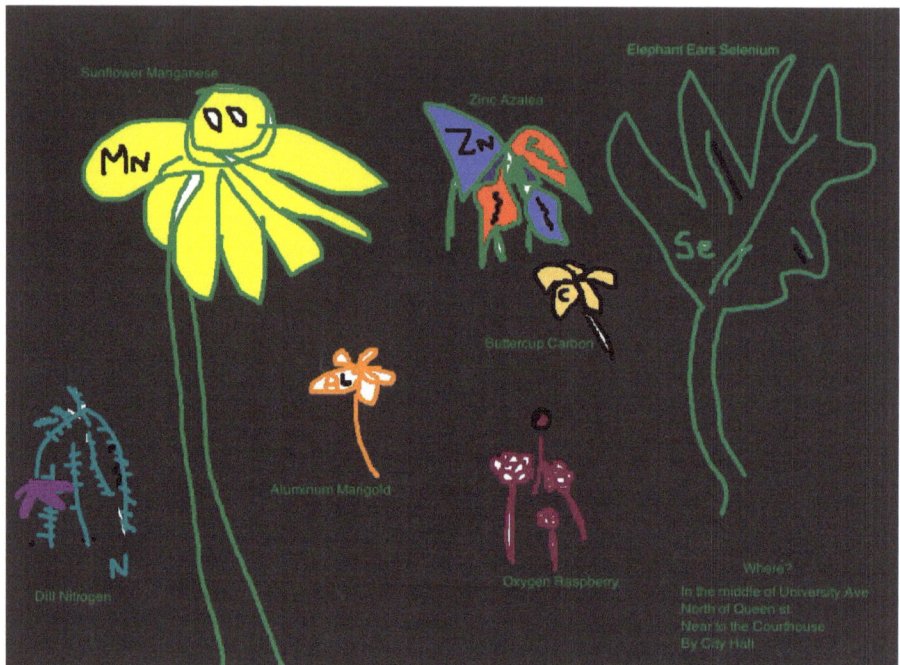

In the middle of University Avenue in Toronto, North of Queen street, near to the Courthouse, by City Hall, someone has planted some wonderful wonderful plants & flowers...It is a giant garden paradise, in the middle of the road, with cars flowing on either side...

Here are some of the flowers & plants that were there with their associated element...

If you know the element a flower contains, then you can plant according to your biochemical needs...

For example, if you are low in Oxygen because you have Liver troubles, you could plant raspberry bushes for the Oxygen...

Sunflower Manganese

Dill Nitrogen

Aluminum Marigold

Buttercup Carbon

Oxygen Raspberry

Zinc Azalea

Elephant Ear Selenium...

www.ingramcontent.com/pod-product-compliance
Lightning Source LLC
Chambersburg PA
CBHW040903180526
45159CB00010BA/2913